Anxiety Disorders Comorbid with Depression

Acknowledgements: Professor Stein is supported by the Medical Research Council of South Africa.

Anxiety Disorders Comorbid with Depression:

Social anxiety disorder, post-traumatic stress disorder, generalized anxiety disorder and obsessive–compulsive disorder

Dan J Stein
Director MRC Unit on Anxiety Disorders
University of Stellenbosch
Cape Town
South Africa
and
Research Associate Professor
University of Florida
Gainesville
Florida, USA

Eric Hollander
Department of Psychiatry
Mt. Sinai School of Medicine
New York
USA

MARTIN DUNITZ

© 2002 Martin Dunitz Ltd, a member of
the Taylor & Francis group

First published in the United Kingdom
in 2002 by
Martin Dunitz Ltd
The Livery House
7–9 Pratt Street
London NW1 0AE

Tel: +44 (0)207 482 2202
Fax: +44 (0)207 267 0159
Email: info.dunitz@tandf.co.uk
Website: http://www.dunitz.co.uk

A CIP record for this book is available
from the British Library.

ISBN 1-84184-050-5

Distributed in the USA by:
Fulfilment Center, Taylor & Francis, 7625 Empire Drive, Florence, KY 41042, USA
Toll free Tel: +1 800 634 7064   E-mail: c serve@routledge_ny.com

Distributed in Canada by:
Taylor & Francis, 74 Rolark Drive, Scarborough, Ontario, M1R 4G2, Canada
Toll free Tel: +1 877 226 2237   E-mail: tal_fran@istar.ca

Distributed in the rest of the world by:
ITPS Limited, Cheriton House, North Way, Andover, Hampshire, SP10 5BE, UK
Tel: +44 (0) 1264 332424   E-mail: reception@itps.co.uk

Printed and bound in Italy by Printer Trento S.r.l.

Contents

Preface   *vii*

Comorbidity   *1*

Symptoms/epidemiology   *12*

Psychobiology   *29*

Treatment   *43*

References   *56*

Index   *69*

Preface

Comorbidity is sometimes seen as a rather dry concept, and one that exists only because our diagnostic systems in psychiatry remain rather awkward. In this book we argue that comorbidity is a key tool for understanding the mood and anxiety disorders. Depression and the anxiety disorders are among the most prevalent and costly of the psychiatric disorders, and it is crucial to advance our understanding of their psychobiology and treatment.

In the first chapter of this volume, we explain why comorbidity is so important a conceptual tool. In the second chapter, we consider diagnostic overlaps and distinctions in depression and anxiety disorders, and review the epidemiology of their comorbidity. The third chapter of the volume focuses on the psychobiology of depression and anxiety disorders, and a final chapter focuses on treatment.

This volume will focus in particular on social anxiety disorder (social phobia), post-traumatic stress disorder, generalized anxiety disorder and obsessive–compulsive disorder. (We have used the term 'social anxiety disorder' rather than 'social phobia' in view of a growing consensus that the former label more accurately reflects the pervasive and impairing symptoms of this condition.) A companion volume by Professor Nutt and colleagues focuses on the comorbidity of depression and panic disorder.

Throughout the volume we highlight the clinical implications of the data that are reviewed. Ultimately, the value of current research on the epidemiology, psychobiology and treatment of comorbid depression and anxiety disorders lies in the implications of this work for the management of our patients. This book is aimed at the practising clinician, and we hope that it will prove to be of practical use.

Dan J Stein
Eric Hollander

Comorbidity

Comorbidity as a key concept

The diagnostic system of modern psychiatry is simultaneously a major advance and a crucial weakness. On the one hand, the development of operational criteria for psychiatric disorders has allowed clinicians to make diagnoses with a reliability that is as impressive as that in other areas of medicine. Furthermore, such criteria have fostered a range of fundamental research, beginning with epidemiological surveys showing the prevalence and costs of mental illness.

On the other hand, there is disappointingly little evidence of the validity of our diagnostic systems. Neurobiological dysfunctions often seem to be shared across different diagnostic entities, and particular psychopharmacological interventions are useful in a spectrum of psychiatric conditions. To advance the psychobiology of psychopathology, it may be necessary to focus on the neurobiology of particular functions (e.g. concentration) which are abnormal in a range of different conditions (e.g. anxiety and mood disorders).

Thus, modern psychiatry has made tremendous advances, but at the same time has far to go before it can lay claim to being a truly mature clinical science. We can

Before DSM-III, e.g.'anxiety neurosis'
    Low reliability
    Low validity

DSM-III, DSM-IV, e.g. 'generalized anxiety disorder'
    High reliability
    Low validity

DSM-?, e.g. 'anxiety associated with psychobiological markers x, y, z'
    High reliability
    High validity

Table 1
Reliability and validity in psychiatric nosology

offer reliable diagnoses, good estimates of prevalence and effective treatments. On the other hand, there are many who hold that existing diagnostic systems have hindered progress in understanding the pathogenesis of psychiatric disorders – further advances will require new approaches to classifying symptoms and disorders (van Praag et al 1990) (Table 1).

One concept that highlights both the strengths and weaknesses of current diagnostic systems is that of comorbidity (Feinstein 1970). The high prevalence of comorbidity in psychiatric patients indicates that psychiatric disorders are not non-overlapping constructs, each associated with mutually exclusive psychobiological dysfunctions. The fact that personality-disordered patients are likely to have several different personality disorders, for example, suggests that these entities and their underlying mechanisms overlap in crucial ways.

The availability of reliable diagnostic criteria, however, allows a careful assessment of the range of comorbidities seen in the community and in the clinic, and these data may well shed crucial light on the complex psychobiology of psychiatric disorders (Robins 1994). Data on which symptoms and disorders are most likely to co-occur, and about the temporal relationships between them, can be used to develop and test different hypotheses about the pathogenesis of psychiatric disorders.

In this volume, we use the concept of comorbidity as a tool that allows for an exploration of major depression (major depressive disorder) and the anxiety disorders. Depression and the anxiety disorders are not only among the most common of the psychiatric disorders (Kessler et al 1994), but are also among the most costly to society (Greenberg et al 1999). Fortunately, there have been major advances in our understanding of the psychobiology and treatment of these conditions. By exploring the comorbidity of depression and anxiety disorders, this volume aims to shed light on their pathogenesis and to provide a rationale for planning treatments.

Depression and anxiety disorders

Depression and the anxiety disorders are among the most common psychiatric conditions, although perhaps no single anxiety disorder is as common as depression itself. Several landmark epidemiological studies support such a conclusion. Thus, in the Epidemiological Catchment Area (ECA) study in the USA, lifetime prevalence of depression was 5.8%, whereas lifetime prevalence for anxiety disorders was 14.6% (Regier et al 1988). In the World Health Organization's (WHO) primary care study, the prevalence of depression and anxiety disorders was 10.4% and 10.5% respectively (Sartorius et al 1996).

Furthermore, depression and anxiety disorders are frequently comorbid. Of patients with lifetime depression, prevalence of a lifetime anxiety disorder is high (47% in the ECA – Regier et al 1998; 58% in the National Comorbidity Survey [NCS] – Kessler et al 1996; and 57% in an earlier meta-analysis – Clark 1989). The likelihood of a particular anxiety disorder co-occurring with depression reflects the base-rate prevalence of that disorder. In all cases, however, the odds ratio (OR) for comorbidity far exceeds co-occurrence simply as a result of base rates (OR = 2.9 for social anxiety disorder, 4.0 for panic disorder and post-traumatic stress disorder, 6.0 for generalized anxiety disorder, with mean OR = 4.2) (Kessler et al 1996).

Although pure anxiety without depression is more common than pure depression without anxiety (Alloy et al 1990), the prevalence of depression in anxiety disorders is still high: 56% in the meta-analysis (Clark 1989). Rates of depression vary depending on the particular anxiety disorder diagnosis, but in general the anxiety disorders are as comorbid with depression (OR = 6.6) as they are among themselves (OR = 6.2) (Kessler 1997).

Similarly, in a study of a psychiatric clinical sample, more than half of the depressed patients had an anxiety disorder, and of these, half had more than one (Zimmerman et al 2000a). In primary care samples, comorbidity of mood and anxiety problems appears to be more common than either disorder alone (Stein et al 1995, Goldberg 1999).

High comorbidity of mood and anxiety disorders in epidemiological and/or clinical samples is also seen in children and adolescents (Angold and Costello 1993, Clark et al 1994), the postpartum period (Stuart et al 1998) and elderly people (Flint 1994, Beekman et al 2000). There is also remarkably high comorbidity of anxiety disorders in bipolar and psychotic mood disorders (Cassano et al 1999, Perugi et al 1999), and anxiety may be a distinguishing feature of mixed bipolar states (Myers and Thase 2000). Finally, it should be noted that anxiety and depression also show extensive comorbidity with other psychopathology (Mineka et al 1998).

Although psychiatric nosologies have traditionally differentiated between depression and anxiety disorders, some authors ('lumpers') have used such data to argue that these conditions represent a single underlying dimension, or that they can be subsumed on an affective spectrum of disorders (Mineka et al 1998). An alternative proposal from some ('splitters') has been to argue for a new diagnostic category – mixed anxiety–depression (Moras et al 1996). This diagnosis is listed in the appendix of the *Diagnostic and Statistical Manual of Mental Disorders*, 4th edn (American Psychiatric Association 1994) on disorders requiring further study, and is included in the *International Classification of Mental and Behavioural Disorders*, 10th revision (WHO 1992).

Ultimately, a theoretical resolution to the debate between 'lumpers' and 'splitters' may not be possible – after all, nature is not 'carved at her joints.' From a practical perspective, however, there is persuasive phenomenological evidence of comorbidity of depression and the anxiety disorders, but also for differences between the two. Similarly, at a psychobiological level there is likely to be some degree of both continuity and discontinuity between depression and the anxiety disorders.

In the psychological literature, a useful distinction has been made between two basic dimensions of affect: positive and negative (Tellegen 1985). A two-factor model has been proposed in which *negative affect* is a non-specific dimension common to both depression and anxiety, whereas *positive affect* is a specific factor related (inversely) to depression. Three-factor models have also been proposed in which *physiological hyperarousal* is included as specific to anxiety (Clark and Watson 1991) or to panic (Barlow et al 1996).

Indeed, three-factor models have obtained empirical support in a number of studies. Reviewing this literature, Mineka et al (1998) propose that *negative affect* is a high-order dimension shared by both depression and the anxiety disorders. Absence of *positive affect* is seen in depression, while *anxious arousal* or *somatic anxiety* is associated with panic, and other components are responsible in other anxiety disorders. These dimensions appear to hold true in children and adolescents. There may also be some physiological support for this kind of dimensional approach (see later, page 35).

Different explanations of comorbidity

Methodological issues significantly affect the degree to which comorbidity is found; the increased prevalence of comorbidity in clinical rather than community settings is known as Berkson's (1946) bias, and the use of structured interviews results in apparently higher comorbidity (Frances et al 1990). Apart from such considerations, there are several possible approaches to understanding the fact that comorbidity of the mood and anxiety disorders is higher than that expected by chance alone (Kaplan and Feinstein 1974, Maser and Cloninger 1990).

Sequence of comorbid mood and anxiety

An immediate question raised by these considerations is the sequence of comorbidity in mood and anxiety disorders. If these are consequences of one another, then what is their temporal relationship – which causes which?

It turns out that anxiety far more commonly precedes depression than vice versa, and that particular episodes of depression may begin with anxiety symptoms (Alloy et al 1990). Temporal relations vary, however, between anxiety disorders; social anxiety disorder and simple phobia are more likely to precede depression and they do so by many years, whereas other anxiety disorders more commonly begin at the same time as or after depression

(Kessler et al 1996, Schatzberg et al 1998). Temporal relationships of anxiety disorders and depression do not seem to differ in early onset versus late-onset depression, although comorbid social anxiety disorder and simple phobia may be more common in early onset depression (Alpert et al 1999).

In the ECA, the average length of any lifetime anxiety disorder was 16 years and that for major depression was 23 years (Regier et al 1998). Nevertheless, in the NCS, almost 83% of patients with a lifetime anxiety disorder reported that one of these was their first disorder, whereas about 44% of those with a mood disorder reported that it was their first disorder (Kessler 1997). In clinical samples, it may be possible to obtain a history of childhood separation anxiety preceding later depression (Kovacs et al 1989, Yeragani et al 1989).

What kind of underlying causal mechanisms might explain the usual sequence of anxiety followed by depression? A range of explanations has been offered, from the biological to the ethological to the cognitive (Table 2).

---

1 Biological

Dysfunction in gamma-aminobutyric (GABA) systems mediates anxiety, and may ultimately lead to changes in monoamine systems and depression (Roy-Byrne and Katon 1997).

2 Ethological

After maternal separation, infant primates show protest (a prototype of anxiety) and then later on despair (a protype of depression) (Bowlby 1980).

3 Cognitive

Anxiety involves early uncertain helplessness in the face of stressors; depression sets in only after hopelessness becomes apparent (Beck 1967).

Table 2
Different explanations for the sequence anxiety-to-depression

These different explanations can perhaps complement one another. They are unlikely, however, to be entirely comprehensive given the variations between individuals and between anxiety disorders. We discuss these issues in more detail in the chapter on psychobiology. There is, however, also a clear clinical message: patients with anxiety disorders deserve early and rigorous treatment. Future research to demonstrate the efficacy of such preventive intervention would be very useful.

Impact of comorbidity

Comorbidity of depression and anxiety disorders has important clinical implications. In particular, comorbidity of depression and anxiety has been associated with significant morbidity, as measured by a range of different indicators, in psychiatric, primary care and community studies (Table 3). Indeed, in this area, the concepts of comorbidity and severity are closely linked (Mineka et al 1998).

In a systematic review of the outcome of anxiety and depressive disorders, for example, Emmanuel et al (1998)

More severe symptoms

More chronic illness

Decreased psychosocial function

Increased work absenteeism

Increased treatment seeking

Greater suicide potential

Greater refractoriness to treatment

From Angst (1993), Bronisch and Wittchen (1994), Brown et al (1996), Clayton et al (1991), Coryell et al (1992), Emmanuel et al (1998), Gaynes et al (1999), Kendall et al (1992), Kessler et al (1994), Levitt et al (1993), Lewinsohn et al (1995), Pawlak et al (1999), Sartorius et al (1996), Shafii et al (1998), Tollefson et al (1993).

Table 3
Impact of comorbidity of depression–anxiety

1 Artefact

The symptoms of depression and anxiety, by definition, show some overlap (Clark 1989), perhaps particularly in children (Brady and Kendall, 1992). An important clinical take-home message is that all patients with depression should be assessed for anxiety and vice versa. On the other hand, a closer examination of the defining symptoms of mood and anxiety disorders also indicates a number of distinctions. This is supported by studies showing different affect dimensions in clinical populations (Mineka et al 1998).

2 Causality

It might be argued that mood and anxiety disorders are risk factors for one another (prognostic comorbidity), or that they are secondary consequences of one another (pathogenic comorbidity). Several studies have demonstrated that certain anxiety disorders often precede major depression (e.g. social anxiety disorder precedes major depression). In this case, the secondary disorder reflects a complication of the primary one. An important clinical message of this argument is the need for early and intensive treatment of psychiatric disorders, so as to prevent secondary comorbidity.

3 Extraneous

It might be argued that extraneous factors underlie both depression and anxiety disorders. A number of studies have argued for a link between early childhood trauma and the later development of mood and anxiety disorders. Also, there is growing interest in the genetic underpinnings of psychopathology – particular genes may constitute a risk factor for the later emergence of depression and anxiety disorders. This kind of work, on both biological and psychological factors, may ultimately lead to novel approaches to the treatment of depression and anxiety disorders.

Table 4
Explanations of depression–anxiety comorbidity

found eight studies that met criteria for inclusion. There was strong evidence that patients with a dual diagnosis had a worse prognosis than patients with a diagnosis of anxiety or depression alone (and some evidence that anxiety disorders have a worse outcome than depressive ones). Similarly, in comparison to patients with non-anxious depression, those with anxious depression may have a poorer outcome and treatment response (Clayton et al 1991, Coryell et al 1992).

A worse prognosis in depressed patients with comorbid anxiety disorders may reflect physician non-recognition, inadequate treatment or non-compliance (Roy-Byrne 1999). Certainly there is evidence that, in a primary care setting, physicians are more likely to recognize depression than anxiety (Ormel et al 1991). Patients with comorbid anxiety may be more likely to be prescribed benzodiazepines than antidepressants (Wittchen et al 1999), and even when prescribing antidepressants physicians may not be aware that anxiety disorders require lower starting doses and longer treatment duration. Depressed patients with comorbid anxiety are more likely to be non-compliant (Brown et al 1996). Finally, the characteristics of the health-care system (e.g. insufficient time) may impact negatively on patients with comorbidity.

Certainly, all patients who present for treatment of depression or anxiety disorders should be comprehensively assessed to determine whether comorbid disorders and symptoms are also present, e.g. identification of comorbid anxiety disorders and symptoms helps to target patients requiring more aggressive treatment for depression. Comorbidity also influences the choice of specific intervention, with more broad-spectrum agents and techniques being preferable (Table 5).

- Mood and anxiety disorders are among the most common of the psychiatric disorders, and they have a comorbidity that is greater than that expected by chance
- Comorbidity is a construct that reflects the strengths (increasing reliability) and weaknesses (incomplete validity) of current diagnostic systems in psychiatry
- Comorbidity of mood and anxiety disorders, if not simply artefactual, reflects a sequence from one to the other, or a consequence of other underlying psychobiological factors
- Anxiety precedes depression more commonly than vice versa; this is seen not only in a given episode with anxiety and depressive symptoms, but also in the relationship of a number of anxiety and mood disorders
- Comorbidity of mood and anxiety disorders has been associated with significant negative impact; it is an important clinical marker that deserves early, rigorous and broad-spectrum interventions

Table 5
Comorbidity take-home messages

In this chapter we review the clinical symptoms of major depression (major depressive disorder) and the main anxiety disorders, focusing on their overlap as well as on important distinctions between them. In particular, we consider issues of differential diagnosis and clinical assessment. In addition, we briefly review studies of epidemiology, demographics and clinical course. In each section, we begin by outlining clinical features and go on to consider comorbidity.

Major depression

Clinical features

The signs of major depression comprise a lowering of mood and a loss of pleasure (anhedonia). These core symptoms are accompanied by a range of psychological and physical complaints. Psychological symptoms include thoughts of worthlessness, excessive guilt and thoughts of death. Physical complaints include changes in appetite, abnormalities of sleep and loss of energy.

The symptom of anhedonia is perhaps fairly specific to depression. Although the neurobiology of anhedonia is not well understood, it presumably reflects dysfunctions that could potentially be used to distinguish depression from other conditions. Psychomotor symptoms in depression may also help differentiate depression from psychiatric comparison groups (Sobin and Sackheim 1997).

In addition, systematic cognitive distortions that overly emphasize negative aspects of the self, the world and the future have been hypothesized as characteristic of depression (Beck 1967). Certainly, cognitive symptoms such as thoughts of worthlessness and hopelessness are useful in making the diagnosis of depression.

On the other hand, some of the physical symptoms of depression appear to be relatively non-specific (Table 5). Insomnia, for example, is seen not only in mood disorders, but also in various anxiety and psychotic disorders. Difficulties in concentration are also present in a range of different disorders such as generalized anxiety disorder and attention deficit hyperactivity disorder.

Depression	Overlap	Anxiety
Depressed mood, anhedonia	Irritability, Apprehension/panic	Hypervigilance, Startle response
Ruminations about past	Negative rumination/worry	Worries about future
Loss of interest	Social withdrawal, Distress, Dysfunction	Agoraphobia
Retardation	Agitation	
Weight gain/loss	Insomnia, Decreased concentration, Chronic pain, Gastrointestinal complaints, Fatigue	

Table 6
Overlap in symptoms of anxiety and depression

Furthermore, withdrawal from social activities and negative thoughts in general are redolent of the avoidance and anxiety concerns that are often seen in anxiety disorders. Avoidance behaviours are characteristic of the anxiety disorders, whereas negative thoughts in depression (rumination) may be redolent of worries (of generalized anxiety disorder), obsessions (of obsessive–compulsive disorder) or other anxiety symptoms.

It is important to distinguish a number of subtypes of major depression. Psychomotor disturbance appears to be a particularly important differentiator of melancholia, perhaps pointing to a unique psychobiology (Parker 2000). Whereas patients with psychomotor retardation are often readily diagnosable as having depression, patients with an agitated depression are sometimes misdiagnosed with an anxiety disorder. In patients with both depression and anxiety, the diagnosis of a bipolar mixed state or bipolar spectrum disorder should also be excluded.

Non-melancholic depression may be approached in various ways too; one distinction that has been made is between 'anxious worriers' and 'irritable/hostile' patients (Parker 2000). Anxious worriers are more likely to have anxiety when depressed, but this distinction is based less on clinical symptoms than on temperament. Thus, 'anxious worriers' are more likely to have a family history of anxiety, to have a history of behavioural inhibition and social anxiety disorder in childhood, to have become dependent on anxiolytic drugs and alcohol, to meet lifetime criteria for an anxiety disorder, to 'act in' when stressed, and to have a cluster C personality style.

Also crucial from the perspective of differential diagnosis are the changes in presentation of major depression in different age groups, e.g. in children and adolescents with major depression, an important symptom is irritability. This symptom is also characteristic of a number of anxiety disorders (generalized anxiety disorder, post-traumatic stress disorder). Children and adolescents with depression may also have symptoms of separation anxiety.

Depression with anxiety

At noted earlier, the prevalence of anxiety disorder in patients with depression has been estimated at 57% in a meta-analysis (Clark 1989), although rates do vary from disorder to disorder. Furthermore, comorbidity of depression and anxiety has been associated with more severe symptoms, worse prognosis, and increased morbidity as measured by a broad range of indicators (see Table 3).

Comorbidity should therefore serve as an important clinical flag. It is crucial to do a thorough evaluation of anxiety symptoms in depressed patients, and to treat such symptoms rigorously. In the next sections, we consider the overlap between depression and each of the major anxiety disorders.

Panic disorder

Clinical features

Panic attacks, although characteristic of panic disorder, may also be seen in a range of other disorders. They are characterized by a discrete period of intense fear or discomfort, with sudden onset and rapid peaking of a range of cognitive and somatic symptoms. Cognitive symptoms include fear of losing control, fear of going crazy and fear of dying. Somatic symptoms reflect activation of the sympathetic nervous system, with consequent cardiac (palpitations, tachycardia), respiratory (shortness of breath, choking feelings), gastrointestinal and oculovestibular symptoms.

Panic attacks in panic disorder are characterized by their spontaneity, coming 'out of the blue'. Thus, although panic attacks in panic disorder may be stimulated by exposure to feared situations (situationally bound or situationally predisposed panic attacks), for the diagnosis of panic disorder the patient must have recurrent unexpected (uncued) panic attacks. Panic attacks may even emerge during sleep – nocturnal panic attacks – a phenomenon that is not often seen in other anxiety disorders.

The particular kind of avoidance seen in panic disorder is also fairly unique. Patients begin to avoid places or situations from which escape may be difficult or in which help may not be available in the event of having panic-like symptoms or a panic attack. This is agoraphobia or, literally, fear of the marketplace. The anxiety typically leads to a pervasive avoidance of a variety of situations, such as being alone outside the home or being home alone, being in a crowd of people, travelling in a car, bus or train, or being on a bridge or in an elevator (American Psychiatric Association 1994).

An important first step in diagnosing panic disorder in the depressed patient, or vice versa, is therefore a careful history focusing on the temporal relationship of panic and depression symptoms. Panic and depressive symptoms differ markedly in their quality, and panic attacks may be followed by depression, or may begin only during the course of a depression (Charney et al 1986).

Panic disorder and depression

Community and clinical studies have indicated that comorbidity of panic disorder and depression, lifetime and current, is perhaps the strongest type of anxiety–mood comorbidity. In the ECA data, the prevalence of these disorders occurring together was 11 times greater than expected by chance (Andrade et al 1994). In the NCS, panic–depression comorbidity was associated with greater symptom severity, chronic course, role impairment, help seeking and suicidality (Roy-Byrne et al 2000).

A range of clinical studies of the comorbidity of panic disorder and depression yields similar conclusions (Johnson and Lydiard 1998, Lecrubier and Uestuen 1998), e.g. in a study of 954 patients with major depression who were followed for 10 years, the presence of panic attacks was one of the strongest predictors of completed suicide within the first year (Fawcett et al 1992). From a clinical perspective, early treatment and careful monitoring of patients with panic–depression is crucial. This subject is covered more fully in the companion volume *Anxiety Disorders Comorbid with Depression: Panic disorder and agoraphobia*.

Social anxiety disorder (social phobia)

Clinical features

The social situations that are feared in social anxiety disorder comprise social interaction and performance situations. Social interaction includes situations such as conversations at work or dating. Performance situations include public speaking, or eating, drinking or writing in front of others. Patients with generalized social anxiety disorder fear most social situations, whereas patients with discrete social anxiety disorder fear only one or a few performance situations.

Like other anxiety disorders, social anxiety disorder is also characterized by avoidance symptoms. Thus, patients avoid social interaction and performance situations, or else endure them with marked anxiety or distress. Such avoidance plays an important role in contributing to the morbidity of social anxiety disorder, e.g. in community surveys, subjects with social anxiety disorder are more likely to be unmarried and unemployed than subjects without social anxiety disorder (Magee et al 1996).

Panic attacks also characterize social anxiety disorder (social phobia). However, the panic attacks of social anxiety disorder have specific elements which allow them to be differentiated from those seen in panic disorder. First, whereas panic attacks in panic disorder are often characterized by dyspnoea, those in social anxiety disorder are more likely to be characterized by blushing, tremor and averted gaze (Amies et al 1983) Second, whereas panic attacks in panic disorder are precipitated by open spaces and other places/situations from which escape is difficult, those in social anxiety disorder are triggered by social situations.

Social anxiety disorder and depression

Social anxiety disorder is associated with a range of other disorders, including major depression, substance use disorders and other anxiety disorders in community surveys (Magee et al 1996, Kessler et al 1999a). Rates of depression in social anxiety disorder are even higher in clinical samples, where social anxiety disorder may precede the major depression in 90% or more of cases, with a lag time of around 13 years (Stein et al 1990). Such data suggest that social anxiety disorder predisposes to the later development of depression and other disorders. Certainly, there is evidence that alcohol abuse in the context of pre-existing social anxiety disorder can be conceptualized as a form of self-medication (Kushner et al 1990).

In the ECA, the risk of suicide-related symptoms in social anxiety disorder occurred primarily in the presence of comorbid depression (Schneier et al 1992). In the NCS, comorbid depression in social anxiety disorder did not increase the risk for a suicide attempt (Kessler et al 1999a), but was associated with higher impairment (Magee et al 1996). In a population-based twin study, a third of adolescents with social anxiety disorder and comorbid major depression had already attempted suicide (Nelson et al 2000). Subjects with social anxiety disorder and comorbid depression were also at elevated risk for alcohol dependence.

Comorbid disorders, particularly mood and other anxiety disorders, are more common in generalized social anxiety disorder disorder than in discrete social anxiety disorder (Kessler et al 1998). Also, depression in social anxiety disorder is often atypical (characterized by hyperphagia, hypersomnia, leaden paralysis and rejection sensitivity). It is possible that generalized social anxiety disorder and atypical depression share certain neurobiological features; the response of both to classic monoamine oxidase inhibitors may be argued to indicate involvement of the dopaminergic system.

Perhaps the most important clinical point to emerge from studies of comorbid social anxiety disorder is the necessity for early diagnosis and treatment. Unfortunately, social anxiety disorder remains under-recognized in primary care practice, with patients presenting for treatment only after the onset of complications such as major depression or substance use disorders (Stein and Chavira 1998). Early and rigorous treatment of social anxiety disorder has the potential to prevent such comorbidity.

Post-traumatic stress disorder

Clinical features

Post-traumatic stress disorder (PTSD) begins by definition in the aftermath of a serious traumatic event, and is characterized by three symptom clusters (Table 7).

A range of symptoms in PTSD is not part of the diagnostic criteria, but is crucial for full understanding of certain patients, and for appropriate intervention. These include symptoms such as shame, guilt and social mistrust. There may also be impulsivity, hostility, dissociation and somatization symptoms. Particularly when traumas begin early in development, and occur multiple times, PTSD may take a complex form, with negative effects on personal relationships, and on affect and impulse modulation (van der Kolk et al 1996).

Table 7
Clusters of symptoms in PTSD. American Psychiatric Association 2000.

Based merely on symptom profile, it can be difficult to differentiate PTSD from depression (which also demonstrates restricted affect, sleep disturbance) (Southwick et al 1991), generalized anxiety disorder (in which there is also hypervigilance, irritability), panic disorder and even obsessive–compulsive disorder (e.g. patients who have been raped may wash themselves repeatedly) (Pitman 1993). Re-experiencing symptoms may be more characteristic of PTSD (Keane al 1997, Blanchard et al 1998, Shalev et al 1998), although depressed patients may report trauma and intrusive traumatic recollections (Carlier et al 2000). The take-home message here is the importance of taking an adequate trauma history in all patients.

Given the overlap of symptoms between PTSD and commonly occurring comorbid conditions, some authors have suggested that these should not be seen as separate, but as 'complex somatic, cognitive, affective and behavioral effects of psychological trauma' (van der Kolk et al 1996). Alternatively, it has been suggested that patients with

PTSD over-report various symptoms in comparison to patients with psychiatric disorders, resulting in artefactually increased comorbidity (Hyer et al 1987). As in other anxiety disorders, however, comorbidity in PTSD comprises a potentially useful tool for investigating subtyping and pathogenesis, and for considering appropriate treatment.

PTSD and depression

Although PTSD is a highly prevalent disorder, it should be remembered that the prevalence of exposure to trauma is even higher. Indeed, PTSD can be characterized as a dysfunctional response to trauma, in which there is a failure to respond adaptively once the threat has been removed (Yehuda and McFarlane 1995). Risk factors for developing PTSD include severity of the trauma, previous exposure to trauma and, in some studies, previous depression (Brady et al 2000).

Furthermore, the assumption that trauma leads specifically to PTSD may be questioned; trauma may result in an adjustment disorder, in depression (Kendler et al 1999) or in a brief psychotic reaction. Repeated traumas during childhood may foster the development of particular personality disorders (e.g. borderline personality disorder). Alternatively, PTSD may itself lead to other comorbid disorders, e.g. substance use disorders may begin in an attempt to self-medicate for PTSD symptoms.

In the NCS, around 48% of PTSD subjects had lifetime major depression, making it the most common comorbid diagnosis (Kessler et al 1995). Similar or higher rates are found in clinical samples (Shalev et al 2000). Depression after trauma is particularly common in those with previous depression and in those who develop PTSD (McFarlane 1989, Shalev et al 1998). Conversely, in some studies comorbid depression appears to predict the chronicity of PTSD (Breslau et al 1991, McFarlane and Papay 1992). Certainly, patients with PTSD and depression are more distressed, have more role impairment and (importantly from a clinical point of view) are more likely to report suicidal ideation (Brady et al 2000).

Although several studies have found that depression is typically temporally secondary to PTSD (Kessler et al 1995), some studies dispute this finding (Shalev et al 2000). Furthermore, there may be differences in the psychobiological mechanisms that mediate early PTSD and depression (see next chapter). It seems reasonable to suggest that PTSD and depression may be independent sequelae of traumatic events, and interact to increase distress and dysfunction (Shalev et al 1998). Different types of trauma may conceivably have different effects on PTSD comorbidity (Deering et al 1996).

Again, an important take-home message is that all patients with major depression should be asked about trauma; indeed, there may be an association between severity of depression and intrusive memories of the trauma (Carlier et al 2000). A second clinical take-home message is that early treatment interventions in PTSD should target both PTSD and depression. The use of benzodiazepines in the aftermath of trauma does not appear to be helpful, and may even exacerbate PTSD symptoms (Gelpin et al 1996). In contrast, antidepressant agents are more likely to target both PTSD and depression symptoms.

Generalized anxiety disorder

Clinical features

In DSM-III, generalized anxiety disorder (GAD) was conceptualized as a 'residual' diagnosis – it was diagnosed only in the absence of other axis I disorders. Indeed, several authors have argued that GAD should not be diagnosed in the presence of a mood disorder (Clayton et al 1991). An alternative perspective on GAD, however, argues that GAD should be seen as a 'basic' anxiety disorder (Brown and Barlow 1992), with the psychobiological processes that mediate GAD serving as vulnerability factors for the development of a range of psychiatric disorders.

It is worth noting, however, that, despite the high comorbity of GAD in many studies, the odds ratios for GAD occurring with other disorders are not unusually high. Indeed, lifetime and episode comorbidities of GAD and major depression are similar, refuting the argument that major depression is a true independent disorder in contrast to GAD (Kessler et al 1999b).

Perhaps the term 'generalized anxiety' contributes to our difficulty in viewing GAD as an independent disorder. It may be useful to see this condition as a 'tension disorder'. Such tension is both psychological (worries, irritability) and somatic (muscle tension, feeling keyed up). This set of symptoms is often primary with depression a later development (Akiskal 1985), but in other cases it is seen as concurrent with, or temporally secondary to, other conditions.

GAD and depression
Comorbidity between GAD and major depression is particularly strong, e.g. in the NCS, subjects with current GAD frequently also had current major depression (39%) or dysthymia (22%) (Kessler et al 1996). Similarly, in GAD patients with a lifetime psychiatric diagnosis, there was often a history of major depression (62%) or dysthymia (39%). Unipolar disorders were four times more common than bipolar disorders (Judd et al 1998). GAD and depression commonly begin within the same year.

Similarly, in the Harvard Brown Anxiety Research Project (HARP) study of a primary psychiatry setting, 54% of GAD patients had either current major depression or dysthymia (Massion et al 1993). Conversely, a number of primary care studies have shown that 35–50% of patients with current major depression have comorbid GAD (Roy-Byrne and Katon 1997); this is often higher than levels of other comorbid disorders.

Comorbidity of GAD and mood disorders is associated with significant negative impact, in terms of disability and dysfunction (Kessler et al 1996). Methodological limitations of such work include the possibility that mood disorders distort perception of role functioning (Kessler et al 1999b). Nevertheless, in the NCS, 28% of pure generalized anxiety respondents reported that symptoms interfered with life activities, in contrast to 51% of respondents with comorbid GAD (Wittchen et al 1994). Conversely, major depression comorbid with GAD is associated with more impairment than major depression without GAD (Kessler et al 1996).

In another analysis of the NCS data, together with the Midlife Development in the US survey, Kessler and colleagues (1999b) emphasized that comorbid major depression and GAD are associated with more impairment than pure major depression or pure GAD. Furthermore, the degree of impairment of pure GAD and pure major depression was similar, providing additional support to the argument that GAD is an important independent disorder, irrespective of whether subjects have comorbidity (Kessler et al 1999b). Similar findings have also been reported in primary care studies (Sherbourne et al 1996, Maier et al 2000).

Comorbidity may also impact on medical utilization. Although GAD is the least common anxiety disorder in mental health-care settings, it is the most common anxiety disorder in primary care settings (Maier et al 2000) and in patients with chronic medical disorders (Sherbourne et al 1996). In the NCS, for example, individuals with comorbid GAD were more likely to seek professional or psychiatric help, and to take medications for GAD symptoms, than those with pure GAD (Wittchen et al 1994, Judd et al 1998).

Notably, patients who present to primary care practitioners with somatic complaints appear less likely to have psychiatric conditions recognized than patients who present with psychosocial problems (Kirmayer et al 1993). Furthermore, anxiety symptoms may be more commonly missed than depressive symptoms (Ormel et al 1991). Given the importance of somatic symptoms in GAD, it is possible that the psychic component of this disorder is often missed. This might result in unnecessary medical consultations and diagnostic tests (Carter and Maddock 1992); indeed, annual medical expenditures for anxious patients have been quoted as being up to 10 times higher than for non-anxious patients (Sherbourne et al 1996).

As for other anxiety disorders, comorbidity may have negative implications for the course of the disorder. Thus, Angst and Vollrath (1991) found that the best predictors of negative course in GAD were severity and duration of symptoms, as well as comorbidity with depression. Similarly, in the HARP study, the likelihood for remission of GAD and any other comorbid condition after 1 year was half the annual remission rate for GAD alone (Yonkers et al 1996). Furthermore, comorbidity of GAD and depression has predicted a poorer response to both pharmacotherapy and psychotherapy (Brown et al 1996; Durham et al 1997). The take-home message again is that comorbidity demands earlier, more rigorous and broader-spectrum intervention.

Obsessive–compulsive disorder

Clinical features
Obsessive–compulsive disorder (OCD) is characterized by intrusive thoughts (obsessions) that increase anxiety, and ritualistic behaviours or mental acts that serve to decrease anxiety. Important symptom subtypes in OCD include those revolving around contamination concerns and washing, other obsessions that require checking,

symmetry and ordering, and hoarding (Leckman et al 1997). A number of OCD patients also have concurrent tics, a distinction that may also have implications for considering underlying psychobiology and appropriate management.

Avoidance symptoms may also be seen in OCD, e.g. patients with contamination concerns and repeated hand-washing may avoid situations in which they may have to face dirt, for fear that they will then need to spend hours washing in order to feel anxiety free. Indeed, the morbidity associated with OCD should not be underestimated – OCD appears to be the tenth most disabling of all medical conditions (Murray and Lopez 1996).

One subtype of OCD that is perhaps particularly relevant to questions of differential diagnosis is obsessional slowness. Such patients may, at first sight, appear to have depression with psychomotor retardation. However, these symptoms in fact reflect intrusive obsessions and repetitive rituals rather than depressed mood. Also relevant here is the subtype of OCD with poor insight; such OCD patients may appear to have delusional disorder or another psychotic condition.

The putative OCD spectrum disorders should also be mentioned in this context (Hollander 1993, Stein and Hollander 1993). Disorders that lie on this spectrum are thought to overlap phenomenologically and psychobiologically with OCD, e.g. body dysmorphic disorder is characterized by repetitive thoughts of imagined ugliness, repeated mirror checking or other rituals, and a selective response to serotonin reuptake inhibitors (Hollander et al 1999).

OCD and depression
Early literature on the relationship of OCD and depression focused on the question of whether OCD was best con-

ceptualized as a mood disorder (Insel 1982). With advances in our understanding of the distinctive psychobiology of OCD, this question has become less relevant. More relevant to current considerations are the implications of comorbid depression for the course and treatment of OCD.

Although OCD commonly precedes major depression, there is also evidence that some patients with major depression are at risk for developing obsessive ruminations (Schatzberg et al 1998). Nevertheless, possible differences between these groups of primary and secondary OCD are not well delineated.

In the ECA, there was evidence that OCD patients with comorbid disorders had certain distinguishing features, such as higher rates of mild cognitive impairment (Hollander et al 1996). Fortunately, however, patients with OCD and comorbid depression respond well to standard OCD treatments (Zitterl et al 2000) (although interestingly, in some cases, a single agent is useful for the OCD but not the depression, and vice versa [Schaller et al 1998]).

- Major depression involves anhedonia and rumination over past events; in contrast, the anxiety disorders are characterized by anxiety and fears about future events
- Nevertheless, depression and anxiety disorders also share certain features, including various somatic symptoms (insomnia, irritability) and distorted cognition
- Panic attacks or symptoms are seen in a number of different anxiety disorders; however, the anxiety disorders are characterized by different kinds of avoidant behaviours
- Depression with anxiety features has negative prognostic implications; this is, therefore, an important clinical marker, which demands early and rigorous intervention
- Similarly, comorbid depression in the anxiety disorders is associated with increased severity and morbidity; early recognition and comprehensive treatment of such comorbidity is therefore crucial

Table 8
Phenomenology take-home messages

Conclusions

Comorbidity of mood and anxiety disorders is common and has significant negative implications for both the course of these disorders and levels of dysfunction. Patterns of depression comorbidity differ across the anxiety disorder, with some variations in temporal relationships; only simple phobia is not associated with major depression. It is important to assess anxiety in patients with depression and vice versa, and it is crucial to initiate early, rigorous and broad-spectrum interventions in patients with comorbidity (Table 8). In patients with single disorders this kind of treatment is potentially important in reducing the risk of later comorbidity.

Psychobiology

If depression and anxiety disorders fall into a spectrum of disorders, an immediate question is the nature of the overlap in their underlying psychobiology. In this section, we explore aspects of the neurochemistry, neuroanatomy and psychology of depression and the anxiety disorders, focusing in particular on continuities and discontinuities across these different conditions. We begin with serotonin, move on to higher level neuroanatomical structures and finally consider psychological schemas.

Neurochemistry

Serotonin

Many different neurochemicals may be involved in both depression and the anxiety disorders. Nevertheless, there is good reason to focus on serotonin in particular, given the importance of serotonergic agents in the treatment of these conditions. Indeed, the efficacy of the selective serotonin reuptake inhibitors (SSRIs) across depression and anxiety disorders raises the question of how such very different disorders can respond to the same class of medication.

A number of different answers have been proposed, and it is worthwhile reviewing these briefly.

First, a see-saw model has been proposed in which serotonin (5-HT) function is low in depression and high in anxiety disorders (Stein and Stahl 2000). This model can be used to explain a number of different findings:

- Animal studies show that a decrease in serotonergic activity is associated with behavioural avoidance
- Gene knock-out studies show that animals with inactivated 5-HT$_{1A}$ receptors (and increased terminal 5-HT) demonstrate anxiety
- *m*-Chlorophenylpiperazine (*m*-CPP), a 5-HT agonist, results in exacerbation of symptoms in a range of anxiety disorders
- During the treatment of anxiety disorder patients with SSRIs there is an initial exacerbation of symptoms; presumably, thereafter, there are compensatory synaptic changes with subsequent decrease in serotonergic activity.

Second, an amygdala model has been proposed in which SSRIs act to increase serotonergic flow, and to switch off an anxiety switch (in anxiety disorder) and to decrease anhedonia (in depression) (Stein and Stahl 2000):

- Animal studies show that an increase in serotonergic activity is associated with a decrease in anxiety
- Gene knock-out studies show that animals with inactivated 5-HT$_{1A}$ receptors (and increased terminal 5-HT) show reduced immobility in antidepressant/stress models
- There are serotonergic circuits that branch to many limbic regions, including the amygdala and its efferents (brain-stem nuclei, periaqueductal grey, hypothalamus). SSRIs result in decreased activation of these structures, including reduced release of noradrenaline from the locus ceruleus and of corticotrophin-releasing factor (CRF) from the hypothalamus.

Noradrenaline

The growth hormone response to administration of cloni-dine, an alpha-2 noradrenergic agonist, is blunted in depression, panic disorder, social anxiety disorder and generalized anxiety disorder (Sullivan et al 1999). However, given the complexity of growth hormone release, and the interdependence of brain systems, it is simplistic to conclude that there is a common noradrener-gic abnormality in these disorders. Indeed, after treatment with SSRIs, there is a significant decrease in 3-methoxy-4-hydroxyphenylglycol (MHPG), consistent with the idea (see above) that these agents may work in part by lower-ing the firing rate of the locus ceruleus (Coplan et al 1997). Catecholaminergic dysfunction may be particularly relevant to comorbid depression in some anxiety dis-orders (Maes et al 1999).

Corticotrophin-releasing factor

In depression, there is increased release of CRF (Nemeroff et al 1984), resulting in increased release of cortisol and downregulation of the glucocorticoid receptor (with non-suppression after dexamethasone) (Holsboer 1988). In post-traumatic stress disorder (PTSD), there is also CRF hypersecretion (Bremner et al 1997), but a decrease in cortisol levels, perhaps reflecting increased glucocorticoid sensitivity (with hypersuppression after dexa-methasone) (Yehuda et al 1991). Interestingly, the hypo-thalamic–pituitary–adrenal (HPA) axis abnormalities in PTSD with comorbid depression resemble those seen in PTSD alone (Yehuda et al 1990).

It has been argued that HPA axis findings in panic dis-order are more reminiscent of PTSD than of major depression (Kellner and Yehuda 1999), e.g. cortisol response on the dexamethasone suppression test appears to fall along the following spectrum: PTSD < panic disorder < normals < major depression. Further-more, there is no increase in cortisol during laboratory-provoked panic attacks. It might therefore be speculated that, in panic disorder, there is also CRF hypersecretion with enhanced glucocorticoid negative feedback.

The reason for enhanced glucocorticoid negative feedback in PTSD, and possibly panic disorder, remains unclear. There may be some genetic predisposition, with low cortisol also being found in family members of PTSD subjects (Yehuda 1999). There is, however, also evidence that a history of past trauma results in decreased cortisol levels in the immediate aftermath of a subsequent rape (Resnick et al 1995).

Of possible relevance to the neurobiology of comorbid anxiety–depression, is that CRF injected directly into the brain in animals results in symptoms that appear to be analogous to both anxiety (startled, fearful) and depression (loss of interest in food or sex). This may be mediated by CRF projections to the locus ceruleus (Butler et al 1990). The locus ceruleus in turn causes release of extrahypothalamic CRF (i.e. from the amygdala and hippocampus) which does not affect the HPA axis, but which does activate the autonomic nervous system directly. Thus, comorbid anxiety–depression may be mediated in part by noradrenergic activity and by amygdala–hippocampal CRF release, with SSRIs being able to reverse activation of both of these pathways.

Neuroanatomy

Basal ganglia

In a series of seminal reviews, Alexander and colleagues (1985, 1986) emphasize the importance of parallel corticortico-striatal–thalamic–cortical (CSTC) circuits in mediating behaviour and behavioural disorders. Disruption of prefrontal circuits to the basal ganglia results in depression, psychomotor disturbance and cognitive impairment.

Certainly, a range of evidence points to the role of the basal ganglia in depression. First, patients with neurological disorders of the basal ganglia often develop depressive disorders. Second, as noted above, psychomotor disturbance is a core feature of melancholic depression. Third, functional brain imaging has demonstrated decreased activity in the basal ganglia in depressed patients (Videbach 2000). Neurosurgery is rarely used in the treatment of depression, but there are nevertheless reports that disruption of CSTC circuits may be useful in refractory patients.

Research on CSTC circuits has also been important in conceptualizing the neuroanatomy of obsessive–compulsive disorder (OCD) (Stein and Hugo in press). Again, several different types of neurological lesions have been associated with OCD symptoms (Table 9). Indeed, early in the last century, an association between basal ganglia lesions and obsessive–compulsive symptoms was noted in patients with postencephalitic parkinsonism. Furthermore, patients with OCD often have tics or increased neurological soft signs. Again, neurosurgical disruption of CSTC circuits has been found useful in refractory OCD.

Imaging studies in OCD have been particularly persuasive in demonstrating involvement of CSTC circuits. Structural imaging studies have been inconsistent, demonstrating a range of findings from reduced to increased basal ganglia

- Infectious/Immune: Postencephalitic Parkinsonism, Sydenham's chorea
- Traumatic/Toxic: Head injury, wasp sting, manganese intoxication
- Vascular/Hypoxic: Infarction, carbon monoxide intoxication, neonatal hypoxia
- Genetic/Idiopathic: Tourette's disorder, Huntington's disease, neuroacanthocytosis

Table 9
Lesions of the basal ganglia associated with obsessive–compulsive disorder

volume in OCD; arguably there is increased volume in the immediate aftermath of streptococcal infection, with shrinkage over time. Functional imaging studies have demonstrated increased basal ganglia activity both at rest and during exposure to a feared stimulus, with reduced activity following both pharmacotherapy and exposure therapy (Rauch and Baxter 1998).

Social anxiety disorder has also been associated with the basal ganglia (Stein and Hugo in press). First, patients who have been treated with dopamine blockers may show an increase in social anxiety. Second, social anxiety is particularly common in patients with Parkinson's disease (and may precede the emergence of motor signs). Third, there is evidence of striatal abnormalities and of reduced striatal dopamine reuptake site densities in social anxiety disorder.

Amygdala–hippocampus circuits

The limbic system is currently conceptualized in terms of two divisions, an orbitofrontal division and a hippocampal division (Table 10). The orbitofrontal division includes the amygdala and several other structures and plays a particularly important role in mediating implicit cognition.

	Orbitofrontal	Parahippocampal
Structures	Amygdala	Hippocampus
Other structures	Infracallosal cingulate	Supracallosal/ posterior cingulate
	Anterior parahippocampus Insula/temporal pole	Posterior parahippocampus Retrosplenium
Function	Implicit processing	Explicit processing

Table 10
Divisions of the limbic system

The hippocampal division includes the hippocampus and plays a particularly important role in mediating explicit cognition.

Consider, for example, the implicit and explicit aspects of an important cognitive–affective process – fear conditioning. Fear conditioning was demonstrated by John Watson, the father of behaviourism, when he demonstrated that little Albert developed a fear of fur-like objects after being presented simultaneously with fur and a loud noise. Although Albert showed fear when subsequently presented with fur-like objects, he was presumably too young to retain an explicit memory of the event that had triggered this fear. Such a process of implicit fear conditioning appears particularly important in understanding the psychobiology of the anxiety disorders.

Preclinical research demonstrates that the amygdala plays a crucial role in implicit fear conditioning. The amygdala receives afferents from the thalamus (external stimuli) and cingulate (response conflict), allowing it early access to information not yet fully processed by the higher cortex, and it has efferents to a range of structures involved in the fear response. Thus, when a feared stimulus is presented, there is automatic (non-conscious) activation of this network.

The hippocampus may play a particularly important role in mediating contextual aspects of fear conditioning, e.g. an animal that has received a series of shocks in a particular cage will subsequently avoid that cage. The explicit memory of this cage is likely to be mediated by the hippocampus. (In infants like little Albert, hippocampal neurons are not yet fully myelinated, so that explicit memory is not well developed.)

These distinctions provide a way of understanding important clinical data. Lesioning of the amygdala may result in the Kluver–Bucy syndrome, which is characterized by attenuated fear responses. In contrast, when the amygdala is hyperactivated, e.g. in seizure disorder, there is increased affectivity/emotionality. Similar kinds of patterns may also be present in subjects who do not have neurological lesions; anxious arousal has been associated with hyperactivation of right parietotemporal regions, whereas low positive affect may be linked to hypoactivation of this area (Heller and Nitschke 1998).

Classically, patients with amnestic disorder secondary to a hippocampal lesion avoid contexts where they have previously experienced negative stimuli, but are unable to articulate explicitly the reason for this avoidance.

Prefrontal cortex
Preclinical data demonstrate that extinction of fear conditioning is mediated by medial prefrontal cortex. It is therefore interesting to note conditions in which the prefrontal cortex is activated (perhaps representing an attempt to extinguish fear responses), and conditions in which there is decreased activity in this region.

Prefrontal activity is increased in OCD and (less so) in GAD (Stein and Hugo in press). Prefrontal activity in OCD is altered by administration of serotonin agonists, and decreases after treatment with SSRIs. In addition, negative affect is associated with increased activity in the right frontal cortex (Mineka et al 1998).

In contrast, prefrontal activity is decreased in depression and impulsivity. Similarly, low positive affect has been associated with hypoactivation of left prefrontal cortex (Mineka et al 1998). Furthermore, there is decreased serotonin transporter binding in the prefrontal cortex of patients with a history of depression, with binding lower in the ventral prefrontal cortex in suicides (Mann et al 2000).

Psychological factors

A classic theoretical distinction is that anxiety is associated with helplessness, whereas depression is characterized by hopelessness (Beck 1967). Indeed, empirical work has indicated that anxiety is associated with anticipated threat, whereas depression is preceded by loss (Brown et al 1993). Furthermore, studies seem to show a reasonable correlation between the different kinds of cognitive distortion in anxiety and depression, and the tripartite model of anxiety–depression symptoms mentioned earlier (preceding chapter) (Mineka et al 1998). There are also some data that patients with comorbid depression and anxiety hold maladaptive beliefs in addition to those typically associated with each disorder alone (Woody et al 1998).

Also relevant to a discussion of the psychological stressors that may precipitate mood and anxiety disorders is work on genetic and environmental contributions to these conditions. Twin studies have suggested that shared genetic factors predispose to major depression and GAD, but environmental factors are also likely to play a role (Kendler et al 1992). Nevertheless, the methodology of this work has limitations (Kessler et al 1999b), and the family history of psychiatric disorders differs in major depression and GAD. Although there may be some genetic overlap between depression and other anxiety disorders (panic disorder, social anxiety disorder), there is also genetic heterogeneity between the anxiety disorders.

Building on the helplessness/hopelessness distinction, differences in negative outcome expectations can be used to conceptualize mixed anxiety–depression. Thus, uncertainty about the ability to control important outcomes may be associated with anxiety, whereas helplessness together with certainty about negative outcome may be associated with depression (Alloy et al 1990). Helplessness together with uncertainty about negative outcome may be associated with mixed anxiety-depression. This view may also explain such aspects of anxiety–depression comorbidity as the typical temporal sequence from anxiety to depression.

Another set of psychological studies differentiates anxiety and depression in terms of cognitive processes. Anxiety involves an attentional bias for threatening information. Thus, when given both threatening and non-threatening cues, anxious patients attend selectively to threatening cues. This takes place without awareness. Anxious patients also show greater anticipation of future negative events (MacLeod and Byrne 1993).

On the other hand, depression involves a memory bias, with depressed subjects showing a bias to recall negative information, particularly when it is self-referential. This occurs during both explicit memory tasks and implicit tasks (when memory is tested indirectly). Depressed patients show not only greater anticipation of future negative experiences, but also reduced anticipation of positive experience (MacLeod and Byrne 1993).

Integrating neurochemistry, neuroanatomy and psychology

The work of Baxter and colleagues (1992) in OCD provides a seminal exemplar for thinking about the mind–brain as a unitary entity. These authors demonstrated that both pharmacotherapy and behavioural therapy resulted in a normalization of activity in CSTC circuits in this disorder. Although there may be differences in the mechanisms on which these two kinds of interventions act, brain and mind are clearly intimately intertwined. Indeed, perhaps rather than speaking about brain and mind, we ought to talk of the brain–mind.

Elsewhere we have argued that the concept of schemas is particularly useful for integrating different perspectives (evolutionary, cognitive, biological) in the mind–brain sciences (Stein 1992). Schemas are cognitive–affective structures which govern the way in which information is assimilated and which, in turn, accommodate the interpretation of this information (Piaget 1952). An evolutionary perspective can be used to supplement a developmental one: to a greater or lesser extent (especially perhaps in higher primates), schemas (which are based in the brain) have evolved in order to optimize behavioural interactions with the world. An immediate question in the context of this volume is the nature of depressive and anxiety schemas, and their overlap.

Depression may have evolved as a mechanism to cope with situations in which ongoing pursuit of a major goal is unlikely to be favourable (Nesse 2000). At a cognitive–affective level, activation of depressive schemas may be associated with an implicit focus on negative memories and altered levels of activity. At a neuronal level, there appears to be dysfunction in prefrontal regions (governing executive functions) and basal ganglia (governing psychomotor symptoms), as well as in the amygdala–hippocampus and their efferents (governing memory and autonomic processes).

What about an anxiety schema? There is in fact likely to be a range of different anxiety schemas; different 'alarms' have evolved in order to respond to different kinds of threat. At a cognitive–affective level, there are different kinds of attentional bias, focusing on different forms of possible harm. At a brain level, these are mediated by somewhat different neurocircuitry, although there may also be shared activation of certain regions across the different anxiety disorders.

Thus, for example, panic disorder may represent a false suffocation alarm (Klein 1993), mediated in part by the amygdala and its efferents (Gorman et al 2000). In PTSD, a similar network is activated, but in addition there may be such elements as deactivation of Broca's area (with decreased verbal processing of traumatic experience) and hippocampal damage (with memory impairment) (Rauch and Baxter 1998). In OCD, on the other hand, there appears to be dysfunction in implicit striatal processing of socioemotional cues, with false activation of evolutionarily based procedural systems (Stein et al 2000). In social anxiety disorder, it has been speculated that there is a false appeasement alarm, perhaps mediated by both striatal and amygdala circuits (Stein and Hugo in press). Serotonergic circuits branch to the various regions that mediate the anxiety disorders, so that treatment with SSRIs results in functional normalization.

Similarly, mixed anxiety–depression may represent the involvement of both depression and anxiety schemas, with mediation by a range of different neuronal circuits, depending on the particular symptoms present. Most studies on the neurobiology of anxiety and depression have focused on unitary disorders, rather than on patients with comorbid conditions. Nevertheless, findings in single disorder studies can presumably be extrapolated, at least in part, to patients with comorbidity. Similarly, there is evidence that patients with comorbid anxiety–depression respond to agents such as the SSRIs. We discuss treatment in greater detail in the next chapter.

In considering schemas (i.e. cognitive–affective structures), it is important also to consider factors that act as schema triggers, e.g. *negative affect* can perhaps be conceptualized as a genetically mediated phenomenon that lowers the threshhold for activation of depressive and anxiety schemas (it appears to involve prefrontal processing, and speculatively is mediated also by the serotonin system). Particular environmental experiences may also selectively activate schemas, e.g. threat/anxiety versus loss/depression.

Indeed, the role of different stressors in precipitating anxiety and mood disorders should not be overlooked. Although trauma is recognized as a defining characteristic in PTSD, it probably also plays an important role in the spectrum of other mood and anxiety disorders. Kraepelin was the first to argue that psychosocial stressors play a greater role in the initial than in subsequent episodes of depressive disorders, and a 'kindling' hypothesis of recurrent depression has received support from a biological (Post 1992), cognitive (Segal et al 1996), and epidemiological (Kendler et al 2000) perspective.

This perspective may be particularly important in considering neurodevelopment. Bowlby's (1980) work on primate isolation was seminal in so far as it successfully

---

- The basal ganglia play a crucial role in mediating depression and obsessive–compulsive disorder; they may also have a role in other disorders such as social anxiety disorder
- The amygdala and its efferents play a crucial role in mediating a fear network, and so may be important in mediating a number of different anxiety disorders
- The hippocampus may play a role in various avoidant/numbing symptoms; it is particularly noteworthy that hippocampal volume is decreased in post-traumatic stress disorder (PTSD)
- Decreased activity in prefrontal cortex may be particularly relevant to impulsive symptoms seen in depression; Broca's area is also decreased in PTSD
- Increased activity in prefrontal cortex is seen in a number of anxiety disorders, including obsessive–compulsive disorder and generalized anxiety disorder; this may reflect activation of a compensatory mechanism
- Serotonergic neurons seem to play a crucial role in mediating symptoms of both anxiety and depression; the selective serotonin reuptake inhibitors (SSRIs) act to normalize mediating circuits in both cases
- Schemas provide one way of integrating several of the different considerations listed here; they may be used to consider evolutionary, cognitive and neurobiological data

Table 11
Neurobiology take-home messages

integrated ethological, affective (psychodynamic) and cognitive perspectives. More recent work has shown that primates traumatized during development have blunted serotonin responses and exaggerated noradrenaline responses (Rosenblum et al 1994) and low cortisol (Coplan et al 1996) as adults. Conversely, social support buffers against depression. Neonatally handled rats show an increased number of glucocorticoid receptors in the hippocampus, enhanced negative feedback and decreased cortisol when stressed in adulthood (O'Donnell et al 1994). Further exploration of such models should allow consolidation of integrated models of mood and anxiety disorders.

Treatment

Psychopharmacology dogma has long indicated that the antidepressants are effective in depression, whereas the benzodiazepines are useful in anxiety. A number of developments have, however, resulted in such dogma being thoroughly overturned. First, the significant problems associated with benzodiazepines have been increasingly appreciated. Second, it has become more and more apparent that certain antidepressants are effective for both the mood and anxiety disorders. In this chapter we review this literature in more detail.

Benzodiazepines

The advantage of the benzodiazepines is that they are quick-acting medications, which rapidly decrease anxiety symptoms. Furthermore, these agents, particularly the high-potency benzodiazepines, have been found to be effective in the treatment of panic disorder and perhaps social anxiety disorder. There is also a small literature on their use in obsessive–compulsive disorder (OCD).

Problems with the benzodiazepines include sedation and dependence, e.g. there is persuasive evidence that patients on benzodiazepines are more likely to be involved in motor vehicle accidents. In addition, the difficulties in discontinuing medication in patients who have

- Sedation/motor vehicle accidents
- Dependence/difficulty in discontinuation
- Interference with exposure therapy
- Association with PTSD emergence
- Disinhibition/paradoxical reactions
- Lack of a broad spectrum effect
- Contraindicated in comorbid substance use

Table 12
Problems associated with benzodiazepine use

been on chronic benzodiazepine treatment should not be underestimated.

The benzodiazepines also theoretically interfere with exposure and response prevention techniques in patients undergoing combined pharmacotherapy and cognitive–behavioural therapy (although admittedly there is relatively little controlled research specifically addressing this issue).

Finally, in the case of traumatized patients, there is a suggestion in the literature (although again the database is limited) that these agents may be associated with emergence of post-traumatic stress disorder (PTSD) (Gelpin et al 1996). Perhaps not dissimilarly, the benzodiazepines have been shown to be problematic in patients with borderline personality disorder, in whom they can cause disinhibition and other negative reactions.

From the viewpoint of comorbidity, perhaps the main problem with the benzodiazepines is the lack of a broad-spectrum effect. Although it has been argued that some benzodiazepines can improve mood, most researchers and clinicians hold that this is not the case. The benzodiazepines may be useful for anxiety symptoms and panic attacks, but for most patients with comorbid mood and anxiety disorders they will not be effective. They are also relatively contraindicated in patients with comorbid substance use disorders.

The benzodiazepines may, however, have a role in the short-term augmentation of antidepressant therapy in anxious depressed or anxiety disorder patients, particularly when high levels of anxiety threaten to disrupt ongoing pharmacotherapy. Controlled trials in depression and anxiety disorders have indicated that the initial combination of an antidepressant with a benzodiazepine may have positive effects, such as reduction of suffering and increased compliance.

Older antidepressants

The tricyclic antidepressants have a distinguished track record in the treatment of major depression, panic disorder and even generalized anxiety disorder (GAD). Although controversial, there is also evidence that these agents are particularly useful in patients with melancholic depression. Furthermore, more recently introduced tricyclic agents can have remarkably good side-effect profiles.

The disadvantage of most tricyclic antidepressants is their relative lack of tolerability. This is perhaps not surprising when one considers the multiple receptors to which the tricyclic antidepressants bind (Table 13); the drugs are not only serotonin and noradrenaline reuptake inhibitors, but also anticholinergics, α_1-adrenergic and α_2-adrenergic agents and membrane-stabilizing compounds. In over-

---

- Serotonin reuptake inhibition
- 5-HT$_2$ blockade
- Noradrenaline reuptake inhibition
- α_1-adrenergic blockade
- α_2-adrenergic blockade
- Acetycholine blockade
- Histamine-1 blockade
- Histamine-2 blockade

Table 13
Receptors at which tricyclic antidepressants act

dose, unfortunately, the tricyclic antidepressants can be lethal.

Furthermore, the spectrum of disorders against which the tricyclic antidepressants (other than clomipramine, a potent serotonin reuptake inhibitor) are effective is limited. Thus imipramine is ineffective for the treatment of social anxiety disorder and OCD, and not a particularly good agent for the treatment of atypical depression. Not all tricyclic antidepressants appear to be useful in PTSD. Also, the tricyclic antidepressants do not have any direct anti-craving effects in patients with comorbid substance use disorders.

The monoamine oxidase inhibitors (MAOIs) have relatively broad-spectrum effects; they are effective in major depression, social anxiety disorder, PTSD, panic disorder and probably GAD. Only their efficacy in OCD is unclear. However, the dietary precautions necessitated by the MAOIs make them impractical as a first-line choice. The reversible inhibitors of monoamine oxidase, (RIMAs) have also been shown to be effective in many of these disorders (depression, social anxiety disorder, PTSD, panic disorder), although many clinicians have questioned the robustness of their effects, and they are not available in the USA.

Newer agents

Newer antidepressant agents include the selective serotonin reuptake inhibitors (SSRIs), the serotonin and noradrenaline reuptake inhibitors (SNRIs), the serotonin antagonist and reuptake inhibitors (SARIs), and the noradrenergic and selective serotonergic antidepressants (NaSSAs). For treatment of anxiety disorders, there is much more information available on SSRIs, and we focus on these. Furthermore, the SNRI venlafaxine is probably primarily an SSRI at lower doses, and the SARIs share serotonin reuptake blockade in common with the SSRIs.

The SSRIs are effective not only in the treatment of major depression, but also in the treatment of each of the major anxiety disorders. Indeed, there is also some information now available suggesting that the SSRIs are selectively effective in certain anxiety disorders (see below). Taken together with their relatively favourable side-effect profile, this broad-spectrum efficacy is persuasive in making the SSRIs first-line agents for the treatment of comorbid mood and anxiety disorders.

The clinical trials database on patients with comorbid disorders is unfortunately relatively sparse. Most trials in psychiatry are designed to exclude subjects with comorbidity; such work may, however, be unrepresentative of clinical settings, where comorbidity is high. Understanding of the mechanisms of therapeutic intervention, together with a knowledge about which agents are effective for which disorders, allow a rational choice to be made when treating patients with comorbid disorders.

In addition, many studies have reported the response of anxious symptoms in depressed patients to the newer antidepressants (Beasley et al 1991, Feighner and Boyer 1992, Moon et al 1994, Fawcett and Barkin 1998, Feighner et al 1998, Flicker and Tsay 1998, Rudolph et al 1998, Silverstone and Ravindran 1999, Sonawalla et al 1999, Versiani et al 1999). Such work provides support for the principle of using these agents as the first line of pharmacotherapy in patients with comorbid depression and anxiety disorders.

SSRIs and other newer agents are better tolerated, and in some studies (Fawcett et al 1995, Zajecka 1996, Lecrubier et al 1997) also more effective than the older tricyclic antidepressants. Furthermore, there are controlled studies demonstrating the efficacy of SSRIs in comorbid OCD–depression (Hoehn-Saric et al 2000), many of the PTSD trials (see below) have included patients with depression and there is a growing interest in trials of comorbid GAD–depression (Goodnick et al 1999).

Current recommendations for the treatment of depression and anxiety disorders increasingly stress the importance of adequate maintenance therapy. Discontinuation of medication during the first year of treatment is associated with an increased risk of relapse. There is a growing database of long-term SSRI trials pointing to the importance of adequate dosage and duration of maintenance treatment. During this phase, it is important to continue to monitor adverse events; weight gain, sleep disturbance, sexual dysfunction or gastrointestinal side effects may contribute to a patient's decision to discontinue medication prematurely.

Other classes of medication

A number of other classes of medication may also be useful in the treatment of complex depression and anxiety disorder cases.

The dopamine blockers may be useful in treatment-resistant major depression as well as in OCD (as augmenting agents). Note, however, that these medications have been associated with an increase in social anxiety symptoms.

The new generation antipsychotics may be particularly useful for a number of reasons. First, they have a better side-effect profile, with reduced risk of tardive dyskinesia, than the older dopamine blockers. Second, they are also $5-HT_2$-receptor antagonists, and this may play a beneficial role in the treatment of comorbid depression and anxiety. Nevertheless, the risk–safety profile of these agents remains relatively disadvantageous.

Anticonvulsants have also increasingly been used in the treatment of mood and anxiety disorders. They are, of course, first-line agents in the treatment of bipolar mood disorder, and they also show efficacy in the treatment of panic disorder, social anxiety disorder, refractory OCD and PTSD. Although there is currently insufficient evidence to list these agents as first line medications in depression and anxiety disorders, they should certainly be considered as augmentation agents in refractory patients. Lithium, although useful in bipolar disorder and refractory depression, has not been shown to be effective in anxiety disorders.

Note that the β-blockers have been mooted as effective in the treatment of discrete social anxiety disorder. It should be emphasized, however, that these agents are not effective for generalized social anxiety disorder, and they may also run the risk of exacerbating depression. Thus, clinicians should arguably have a low threshhold for diagnosing generalized social anxiety disorder, and for initiating an SSRI.

SSRIs in anxiety disorders

Earlier we noted that, in some of the anxiety disorders, the SSRIs are not only effective but are also selectively effective (in comparison with other agents).

Consider, for example, the use of SSRIs in OCD. Classic early work demonstrated that clomipramine, an SRI (serotonin reuptake inhibitor), is more effective than desipramine, a noradrenaline reuptake inhibitor, in OCD. Indeed, each of the SSRIs (selective serotonin reuptake inhibitors) has since been shown to be effective in OCD. Data from the trial of citalopram, the most selective of the SSRIs, is presented in Figure 1 (Montgomery et al 2001). In contrast, there is little evidence that agents without serotonergic actions are useful in this disorder. Interestingly, clomipramine is more effective than desipramine in a range of putative OCD spectrum disorders, including body dysmorphic disorder, trichotillomania and severe nail-biting, as well as for obsessive–compulsive symptoms in autism (Stein 2000a). Similarly, there is evidence for a number of SSRIs for efficacy in such conditions (Joubert and Stein 1999).

Trials with SSRIs in social anxiety disorder are given in Table 14 and in PTSD in Table 15. In the case of social anxiety disorder, there is some evidence that the effect size for the SSRIs is larger than that seen for the RIMAs (van der Linden et al 2000). Similarly, for PTSD there is some evidence that serotonergic agents are more effective than noradrenergic ones (Penava et al 1997).

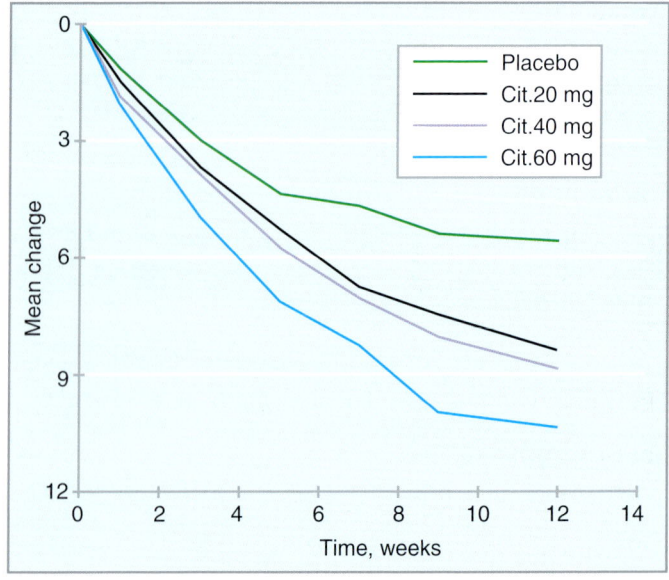

Figure 1
Mean change in Y–BOCS total score, ITT (LOCF) (Reproduced with permission from Montgomery et al 2001.)

Reference	Agent	Drug response	Placebo response
van Vliet et al (1994)	Fluvoxamine	7/15	1/13
Katzelnick et al (1995)	Sertraline	6/12	1/12
Stein et al (1998)	Paroxetine	50/91	22/92
Stein et al (1999)	Fluvoxamine	18/42	10/44
Allgulander et al (1999)	Paroxetine	31/44	4/48
Baldwin et al (1999)	Paroxetine	90/137	47/145
Pfizer	Sertraline	71/134	20/69
SmithKline Beecham	Paroxetine	120/268	26/92
TOTAL		373/701 (53%)	121/471 (26%)

Table 14
Controlled trials of selective serotonin reuptake inhibitors in social anxiety disorder

Reference	Agent	Subjects	Drug response	Placebo response
Amital et al 1999	Sertraline	Predominantly combat-related	15/19	4/23
Brady et al 2000	Sertraline	Predominantly civilian	61/90	44/93
Connor et al 1999	Fluoxetine	Civilian	10/26	4/27
Stein 2000b	Paroxetine	Predominantly civilian	86/143	67/137
Total			172/278 (62%)	129/280 (46%)

Table 15
Controlled trials of selective serotonin reuptake inhibitors in post-traumatic stress disorder (Stein et al 2000b)

- The benzodiazepines should be restricted to use as augmentation agents; although these agents reduce symptoms quickly, their discontinuation is often problematic
- The tricyclic antidepressants are useful for panic disorder and depression, and the monoamine oxidase inhibitors have an even broader profile of efficacy; nevertheless, tolerability issues restrict the use of these agents
- The selective serotonin reuptake inhibitors (SSRIs) have a broad spectrum of activity in the mood and anxiety disorders and are also well tolerated; they are a first-line choice in patients with comorbid depression and anxiety/anxiety disorders
- Dopamine blockers and anticonvulsants may also have a role in the treatment of comorbid depression and anxiety disorders, particularly in treatment-refractory patients
- It is important to use trials of appropriate dose and duration in treating depression and anxiety disorders; maintenance treatment after recovery is also crucial to prevent relapse

Table 16
Treatment take-home messages

In addition, a meta-analysis of trials of SSRIs in panic disorder indicated that the SSRIs are more effective than imipramine and benzodiazepines (Boyer 1995). Consistent with these data, a meta-analysis of trials of nefazodone versus imipramine in depressed patients indicated that, in those with comorbid panic, only nefazodone was more effective than placebo (Zajecka 1996).

There is also growing interest in the use of SSRIs for GAD. An open trial of paroxetine was effective in GAD, and preliminary reports of the placebo-controlled trials of this agent are also positive. Although buspirone and hydroxyzine are effective in some GAD studies (Gale et al 2000), these agents are ineffective in many of the conditions that often accompany GAD (e.g. depression, other anxiety disorders). Venlafaxine has been approved by the US Food and Drug Administration (FDA) for the treatment of GAD; at the doses recommended by the manufacturer, it arguably has primarily serotonergic activity.

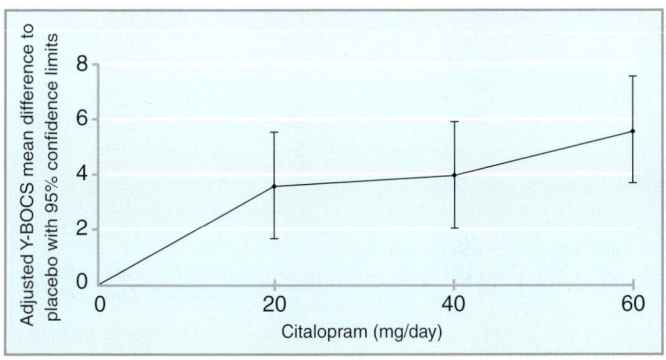

Figure 2
Estimated dose–response relationship after 12 weeks treatment (Repeated measurements ANCOVA, ITT) (Reproduced with permission from Montgomery et al 2001.)

Dose and duration issues

Note that the dose and duration of the SSRIs may differ from disorder to disorder, e.g. it is important to begin the treatment of panic disorder with particularly low doses in order to avoid increased agitation and anxiety. Although dose–response curves with the SSRIs tend to be rather flat, there is some evidence that higher doses are necessary in OCD (Figure 2) (Montgomery et al 2001). Certainly, individual patients with depression or any one of the anxiety disorders may require doses that are higher than usual. Also, patients who relapse during treatment with an SSRI often respond to a further increase in dose.

Patients with major depression, PTSD, GAD or panic disorder are thought to require a trial that is at least 6–8 weeks in duration. There is also some evidence that patients with OCD and social anxiety disorder require trials of longer duration; it is reasonable to treat these disorders for up to 12 weeks before deciding that a particular SSRI is not effective.

Based on these kinds of consideration, it may be suggested that, in patients with comorbid anxiety–depression, particularly when there is evidence of panic symptoms, starting with a relatively low dose of an SSRI is useful. In patients who do not respond, however, it may be necessary to increase doses to maximal levels. Furthermore, a trial should last for 8–12 weeks in order to determine efficacy. Finally, maintenance treatment should be continued for at least a year, and perhaps longer should individual circumstances merit such a decision.

Children and elderly people

There is growing awareness of the prevalence and morbidity of anxiety disorders in both children and older people. Issues of medication tolerability are particularly important in these age groups, so that the SSRIs are again often favoured. Furthermore, there is a growing clinical trials database demonstrating the efficacy and safety of the SSRIs in childhood OCD, PTSD and social anxiety disorder (Hawkridge and Stein 1998, Seedat et al 2001). Although there is less work on anxiety–depression comorbidity itself, it seems reasonable to extrapolate from studies demonstrating the value of SSRIs to the recommendation that these agents should also be a first-line choice in younger and elderly patients with comorbidity.

Psychotherapy

The role of psychotherapy in the treatment of anxiety disorders and depression should not be ignored. Psychoeducation is undoubtedly a key component in the treatment of both. Furthermore, cognitive-behavioural therapy (CBT) in particular has proved useful in many of the anxiety disorders as well as in depression.

As in the case of medication studies, there is a relative paucity of work focusing on comorbidity itself, e.g.

depressed patients may hypothetically be less able to comply with exposure. Still, it would seem reasonable to list CBT as a first-line psychotherapy in the treatment of patients with both anxiety disorders and depression, provided that modifications to standard treatment protocols focusing on single disorders can be made, and noting that a longer course of treatment may be necessary (Woody et al 1999, Menin and Heimberg 2000).

Although there are relatively few studies comparing SSRIs with CBT and combined therapy, clinical experience suggests that the combination of these modalities is often useful. Theoretically, CBT has particular value in preventing relapse after medication discontinuation. In addition, family involvement may be particularly useful in encouraging patients to comply with both medication treatment and exposure exercises.

References

Akiskal HS. Anxiety: Definition, relationship to depression, and proposal for an integrative model. In: Tuma AH, Maser JD, eds, *Anxiety and the Anxiety Disorders*. Hillsdale, NJ: Lawrence Earlbaum Associates, 1985: 787–97.

Alexander GE, DeLong MR. Microstimulation of the primate neostriatum, II: somatotropic organization of striatal microexcitable zones and their relation to neuronal response properties. *J Neurophysiol* 1985; **53:** 1417–30.

Alexander GE, DeLong MR, Strick PL. Parallel organization of functionally segregated circuits linking basal ganglia and cortex. *Annu Rev Neurosci* 1986; **9:** 357–81.

Allgulander C. Paroxetine in social anxiety disorder: A randomized placebo-controlled study. *Acta Psychiatr Scand* 1999; **100:** 193–8.

Alloy L, Kelly K, Mineka S, Clements C. Comorbidity in anxiety and depressive disorders: a helplessness/hopelessness perspective. In: Maser JD, Cloninger CR, eds, *Comorbidity of Anxiety and Mood Disorders*. Washington, DC: American Psychiatric Press, 1990: 499–553.

Alpert JE, Fava M, Uebelacker LA et al. Patterns of axis I comorbidity in early-onset versus late-onset major depressive disorder. *Biol Psychiatry* 1999; **46:** 202–11.

American Psychiatric Association. *Diagnostic and Statistical Manual of Mental Disorders*, 4th edn. Washington, DC: American Psychiatric Press, 1994. (Text revision published 2000.)

Amies PL, Gelder MG, Shaw PM. Social phobia: A comparative clinical study. *Br J Psychiatry* 1983; **142:** 174–9.

Andrade L, Eaton WW, Chilcoat H. Lifetime comorbidity of panic attacks and major depression in a population-based study: Symptom profiles. *Br J Psychiatry* 1994; **165:** 363–9.

Angold A, Costello EJ. Depressive comorbidity in children and adolescents: empirical, theoretical, and methodological issues. *Am J Psychiatry* 1993; **150:** 1779–991.

Angst J. Comorbidity of anxiety, phobia, compulsion and depression. *Int Clin Psychopharmacol* 1993; **8S:** 21–5.

Angst J, Vollrath M. The natural history of anxiety disorders. *Acta Psychiatr Scand* 1991; **84:** 446–52.

Baldwin D, Bobes J, Stein DJ et al. Paroxetine in the treatment of social phobia/social anxiety disorder: Randomized, double-blind, placebo-controlled study. *Br J Psychiatry* 1999; **175:** 120–6.

Barlow DH, Chorpita BF, Turovsky J. Fear, panic, anxiety and disorders of emotion. *Nebr Symp Motiv* 1996; **43:** 251–8.

Baxter LR, Schwartz JM, Bergman KS et al. Caudate glucose metabolic rate changes with both drug and behavior therapy for OCD. *Arch Gen Psychiatry* 1992; **49:** 681–9.

Beasley CM Jr, Sayler ME et al. High-dose fluoxetine: Efficacy and activating-sedating effects in agitated and retarded depression. *J Clin Psychopharmacol* 1991; **14:** 321–7.

Beck AT. *Depression: Clinical, experimental, and theoretical aspects*. New York: Harper & Row, 1967.

Beekman ATF, de Beurs E, van Balkom AJLM, et al. Anxiety and depression in later life: Co-occurrence and communality of risk factors. *Am J Psychiatry* 2000; **157:** 89–95.

Berkson J. Limitations of the application of four-fold tables to hospital data. *Biometric Bull* 1946; **2:** 47–53.

Blanchard EB, Buckley TC, Hickling EJ et al. Posttraumatic stress disorder and comorbid major depression: Is the correlation an illusion? *J Anx Dis* 1998; **12:** 21–37.

Bleich A, Koslowsky M, Dolev A, Lerer B. Posttraumatic stress disorder and depression. *Br J Psychiatry* 1997; **170:** 479–82.

Boyer W. Serotonin uptake inhibitors are superior to imipramine and alprazolam in alleviating panic attacks: a meta-analysis. *Int Clin Psychopharmacol* 1995; **10:** 45–9.

Bowlby J. *Attachment and Loss*, Vol 3. New York: Basic Books, 1980.

Brady EU, Kendall PC. Comorbidity of anxiety and depression in children and adolescents. *J Consult Clin Psychol* 1992; **111:** 244–55.

Brady KT, Killeen TK, Brewerton T et al. Comorbidity of psychiatric disorders and posttraumatic stress disorder. *J Clin Psychiatry* 2000; **61(suppl 7):** 22–32.

Bremner JD, Licinio J, Darnell A et al. Elevated CSF corticotropin-releasing factor concentrations in posttraumatic stress disorder. *Am J Psychiatry* 1997; **154:** 624–9.

Breslau N, Davis GC, Andreski P, Peterson E. Traumatic events and posttraumatic stress disorder in an urban population of young adults. *Arch Gen Psychiatry* 1991; **48:** 216–22.

Bronisch T, Wittchen HU. Suicidal ideation and suicide attempts: comorbidity with depression, anxiety disorders, and substance abuse disorders. *Eur Arch Psychiatry Clin Neurosci* 1994; **244:** 93–8.

Brown C, Schulberg HC, Madonia MJ, Shear MK. Treatment outcomes for primary care patients with major depression and lifetime anxiety disorders. *Am J Psychiatry* 1996; **153:** 1293–300.

Brown GW, Harris TO, Eales MJ. Aetiology of anxiety and depressive disorders in an inner-city population. 2. Comorbidity and adversity. *Psychol Med* 1993; **23:** 155–65.

Brown TA, Barlow DH. Comorbidity among anxiety disorders: Implications for treatment and DSM-IV. *J Consult Clin Psychol* 1992; **60:** 835–44.

Butler PD, Weiss JM, Stout JC et al. Corticotropin-releasing factor produces fear-enhancing and behavioral activating effects following infusion into the locus coeruleus. *J Neurosci* 1990; **10:** 176–83.

Carlier IVE, Voerman BE, Gersons BPR. Intrusive traumatic recollections and comorbid posttraumatic stress disorder in depressed patients. *Psychosom Med* 2000; **62:** 26–32.

Carter CS, Maddock RJ. Chest pain in generalized anxiety disorder. *Int J Psychiatry Med* 1992; **22:** 291–8.

Cassano GB, Pini S, Saettoni M et al. Multiple anxiety disorder comorbidity in patients with mood spectrum disorders with psychotic features. *Am J Psychiatry* 1999; **156:** 474–6.

Charney DS, Heninger GR, Price LH, Breier A. Major depression and panic disorder: Diagnostic and neurobiological relationships. *Psychopharmacol Bull* 1986; **22:** 503–11.

Clark DB, Smith MG, Neighbors BD, Skerlec LM. Anxiety disorders in adolecence: characteristics, prevalence, and comorbidities. Clin Psychol Rev 1994; **14:** 113–37.

Clark LA. The anxiety and depressive disorders: descriptive psychopathology and differential diagnosis. In: Kendall PC, Watson D, eds, *Anxiety and Depression: Distinctive and overlapping features.* San Diego: Academic Press, 1989: 83–129.

Clark LA, Watson D. Theoretical and empirical issues in differentiating depression from anxiety. In: Becker J, Kleinman A, eds, *Psychosocial Aspects of Depression.* Hillsdale, NJ: Erlbaum, 1991; 39–65.

Clayton PJ, Grove WM, Coryell W et al. Follow-up and family study of anxious depression. *Am J Psychiatry* 1991; **148:** 1512–17.

Coplan JD, Andrews MW, Rosenblum LA et al. Persistent elevations in adult nonhuman primates exposed to early-life stressors: implications for the pathophysiology of mood and anxiety disorders. *Proc Natl Acad Sci USA* 1996; **93:** 1619–23.

Coplan JD, Papp LA, Pine D et al. Clinical improvement with fluoxetine therapy and noradrenergic function in patients with panic disorder. *Arch Gen Psychiatry* 1997; **54:** 643–8.

Coryell W, Endicott J, Winokur G. Anxiety syndromes as epiphenomena of primary major depression: outcome and familial psychopathology. *Am J Psychiatry* 1992; **149:** 100–7.

Deering CG, Glover SG, Ready D et al. Unique patterns of comorbidity in posttraumatic stress disorder from different sources of trauma. *Compr Psychiatry* 1996; **37:** 336–46.

Durham RC, Allan T, Hackett CA. On predicting improvement and relapse in generalized anxiety disorder following psychotherapy. *Br J Clin Psychol* 1997; **36:** 101–19.

Emmanuel J, Simmonds S, Tyrer P. Systematic review of the outcome of anxiety and depressive disorders. *Br J Psychiatry* 1998; **173(suppl 43):** 35–41.

Fawcett J, Barkin RL. A meta-analysis of eight randomized, double-blind, controlled clinical trials of mirtazapine for the treatment of patients with major depression and symptoms of anxiety. *J Clin Psychiatry* 1998; **59:** 123–7.

Fawcett J, Scheftner WA, Fogg L et al. Time-related predictors of suicide in major affective disorder. *Am J Psychiatry* 1992; **147:** 1189–94.

Fawcett J, Marcus RN, Anton SF et al. Response of anxiety and agitation symptoms during nefazodone treatment of major depression. *J Clin Psychiatry* 1995; **56(suppl 6):** 37–42.

Feighner JP, Boyer WF. Paroxetine in the treatment of depression: a comparison with imipramine and placebo. *J Clin Psychiatry* 1992; **53(suppl 2):** 44–7.

Feighner JP, Entsuah AR, McPherson MK. Efficacy of once-daily venlafaxine extended release (XR) for symptoms of anxiety in depressed outpatients. *J Affect Disord* 1998; **47:** 55–62.

Feinstein AR. The pretherapeutic classification of co-morbidity in chronic disease. *J Chronic Dis* 1970; **23:** 455–68.

Flicker C, Tsay JY. Citalopram treatment of depression with anxiety. Poster presentation at Biological Psychiatry meeting, Toronto, Canada, May 1998.

Flint AJ. Epidemiology and comorbidity of anxiety disorders in the elderly. *Am J Psychiatry* 1994; **151:** 640–9.

Frances A, Widiger TA, Fyer MR. The influence of classification methods on comorbidity. In: Maser JD, Cloninger CR, eds, *Comorbidity of Anxiety and Mood Disorders.* Washington, DC: American Psychiatric Press, 1990: 41–59.

Gale C, Oakley-Browne M. Anxiety disorder. *BMJ* 2000; **32:** 1204–7.

Gaynes BN, Magruder MM, Burnes BJ et al. Does a co-existing anxiety disorder predict persistence of depressive illness in primary care patients with major depression? *Gen Hosp Psychiatry* 1999; **21:** 158–67.

Gelpin E, Bonne O, Peri T et al. Treatment of recent trauma survivors with benzodiazepines: a prospective study. *J Clin Psychiatry* 1996; **57:** 390–4.

Goldberg D. The management of anxious depression in primary care. *J Clin Psychiatry* 1999; **60(suppl 7):** 39–42.

Goodnick PJ, Puig A, DeVane C et al. Mirtazapine in major depression with comorbid generalized anxiety disorder. *J Clin Psychiatry* 1999; **60:** 446–8.

Gorman JM, Kent JM, Sullivan GM, Coplan JD. Neuroanatomical hypothesis of panic disorder, revised. *Am J Psychiatry* 2000; **157:** 493–505.

Greenberg PE, Sisitsky T, Kessler RC et al. The economic burden of anxiety disorders in the 1990s. *J Clin Psychiatry* 1999; **60:** 427–35.

Hawkridge S, Stein DJ. Risk-benefit assessment of drug therapies for anxiety disorders in children and adolescents. *Drug Safety* 1998; **19:** 283–97.

Heller W, Nitschke JB. The puzzle of regional brain activity in depression and anxiety: The importance of subtypes and comorbidity. *Cognition Emotion* 1998; **12:** 421–47.

Hoehn-Saric R, Ninan P, Black DW et al. Multicenter double-blind comparison of sertraline and desipramine for concurrent obsessive-compulsive and major depressive disorders. *Arch Gen Psychiatry* 2000; **57:** 76–82.

Hollander E. *Obsessive–Compulsive Related Disorders.* Washington, DC: American Psychiatric Press, 1993.

Hollander E, Greenwald S, Neville D et al. Uncomplicated and comorbid obsessive–compulsive disorder in an epidemiological sample. *Depress Anxiety* 1996–7; **4:** 111–19.

Hollander E, Andrea A, Kwon J et al. Clomipramine vs desipramine crossover trial in body dysmorphic disorder: Selective efficacy of a serotonin reuptake inhibitor in imagined ugliness. *Arch Gen Psychiatry* 1999; **56:** 1033–9.

Holsboer F. Implications of altered limbic–hypothalamic–pituitary–adrenocortical (LHPA) function for neurobiology of depression. *Acta Psychiatr Scand* 1988; **77(suppl 341):** 72–111.

Hyer L, Fallon J, Harrison W et al. MMPI overreporting by Vietnam combat veterans. *J Clin Psychol* 1987; **43:** 79–83.

Insel TR. Obsessive compulsive disorder – five clinical questions and a suggested approach. *Compr Psychiatry* 1982; **23:** 241–51.

Johnson MR, Lydiard RB. Comorbidity of major depression and panic disorder. *J Clin Psychol* 1998; **54:** 201–10.

Joubert AF, Stein DJ. Citalopram and anxiety disorders. *Rev Contemp Pharmaco* 1999; **10:** 79–131.

Judd LL, Kessler RC, Paulus MP et al. Comorbidity as a fundamental feature of generalized anxiety disorders: results from the National Comorbidity Survey (NCS). *Acta Psychiatr Scand* 1998; **98(suppl 393):** 6–11.

Kaplan MH, Feinstein AR. The importance of classifying initial comorbidity in evaluating the outcome of diabetes mellitus. *J Chronic Dis* 1974; **27:** 387–404.

Katzelnick DJ, Kobak KA, Greist JH et al. Sertraline for social phobia: a double-blind, placebo-controlled crossover study. *Am J Psychiatry* 1995; **152:** 1368–71.

Keane TM, Taylor KL, Penk WE. Differentiating post-traumatic stress disorder (PTSD) from major depression (MDD) and generalized anxiety disorder (GAD). *J Anxiety Disord* 1997; **11:** 317–28.

Kellner M, Yehuda R. Do panic disorder and posttraumatic stress disorder share a common psychoneuroendocrinology? *Psychoneuroendocrinology* 1999; **24:** 485–504.

Kendall PC, Kortlander E, Chansky TE, Brady EU. Comorbidity of anxiety and depression in youth: treatment implications. *J Consult Clin Psychol* 1992; **60:** 869–80.

Kendler KS, Neale MC, Kessler RC et al. Major depression and generalized anxiety disorder. Same genes, (partly) different environments? *Arch Gen Psychiatry* 1992; **49:** 716–22.

Kendler KS, Karkowski LM, Prescott CA. Causal relationship between stressful life events and the onset of major depresion. *Am J Psychiatry* 1999; **156:** 837–41.

Kendler KS, Thornton LM, Gardner CO. Stressful life events and previous episodes in the etiology of major depression in women: An evaluation of the 'kindling' hypothesis. *Am J Psychiatry* 2000; **157:** 1243–51.

Kessler RC. The prevalence of psychiatric comorbidity. In: Wetzler S, Sanderson WC, eds, *Treatment Strategies for Patients with Psychiatric Comorbidity.* New York: Wiley, 1997; 23–48.

Kessler RC, McGonagle KA, Zhao S et al. Lifetime prevalence and 12-month prevalence of DSM-III-R psychiatric disorders in the United States. *Arch Gen Psychiatry* 1994; **51:** 8–19.

Kessler RC, Sonnega A, Bromet E et al. Posttraumatic stress disorder in the National Comorbidity Survey. *Arch Gen Psychiatry* 1995; **52:** 1048–60.

Kessler RC, Nelson CB, McGonagle KA et al. Comorbidity of DSM-III-R major depressive disorder in the general population: results from the US National Comorbidity Survey. *Br J Psychiatry* 1996; **168:** 17–30.

Kessler RC, Stein MB, Berglund P. Social phobia subtypes in the National Comorbidity Survey. *Am J Psychiatry* 1998; **155:** 613–19.

Kessler RC, Stang P, Wittchen H-U et al. Lifetime co-morbidities between social phobia and mood disorders in the US National Comorbidity Survey. *Psychol Med* 1999a; **29:** 555–67.

Kessler RC, DuPont RL, Berglund P et al. Impairment in pure and comorbid generalized anxiety disorder and major depression at 12 months in two national surveys. *Am J Psychiatry* 1999b; **156:** 1915–23.

Kirmayer LJ, Robbins JM, Dworkind M et al. Somatization and the recognition of depression and anxiety in primary care. *Am J Psychiatry* 1993; **150:** 734–41.

Klein DF. False suffocation alarms, spontaneous panics, and related conditions: An integrative hypothesis. *Arch Gen Psychiatry* 1993; **50:** 306–17.

Kovacs M, Gatsonis C, Paulauskas SL et al. Depressive disorders in childhood. IV. A longitudinal study of co-morbidity with and risk for anxiety disorders. *Arch Gen Psychiatry* 1989; **46:** 776–82.

Kushner MG, Sher KJ, Beitman BD. The relation between alcohol problems and the anxiety disorders. *Am J Psychiatry* 1990; **147:** 685–95.

Leckman JF, Grice DE, Boardman J et al: Symptoms of obsessive–compulsive disorder. *Am J Psychiatry* 1997; **154:** 911–17.

Lecrubier Y, Bourin M, Moon CA et al. Efficacy of venlafaxine in depressive illness in general practice. *Acta Psychiatr Scand* 1997; **95:** 485–93.

Lecrubier Y, Uestuen TB. Panic and depression: A worldwide primary care perspective. *Int Clin Psychopharmacol* 1998; **13(suppl 4):** 7–11.

Levitt AJ, Joffe RT, Brecher D et al. Anxiety disorders and anxiety symptoms in a clinical sample of seasonal and non-seasonal depressives. *J Affect Disord* 1993; **28:** 51–6.

Lewinsohn PM, Rohde P, Seeley JR. Adolescent psychopathology. III. The clinical consequences of comorbidity. *J Am Acad Child Adolesc Psychiatry* 1995; **34:** 510–19.

MacLeod AK, Byrne A. Anxiety, depression, and the anticipation of future postive and negative experiences. *J Abnorm Psychol* 1993; **102:** 238–47.

McFarlane AC. The aetiology of post-traumatic morbidity: predisposing, precipitating and perpetuating factors. *Br J Psychiatry* 1989; **154:** 221–8.

McFarlane AC, Papay P. Multiple diagnoses in posttraumatic stress disorder in the victims of a natural disaster. *J Nerv Ment Dis* 1992; **180:** 498–504.

Maes M, Ai-hua L, Verkerk R et al. Serotonergic and noradrenergic markers of post-traumatic stress disorder with and without depression. *Neuropsychopharmacology* 1999; **20:** 188–97.

Magee WJ, Eaton WW, Wittchen H-U et al. Agoraphobia, simple phobia, and social phobia in the National Comorbidity Survey. *Arch Gen Psychiatry* 1996; **53:** 159–68.

Maier W, Gansicke M, Freyberger HJ et al. Generalized anxiety disorder (ICD-10) in primary care from a cross-cultural perspective: a valid diagnostic entity? *Acta Psychiatr Scand* 2000; **101:** 29–36.

Mann JJ, Huang YY, Underwood MD et al. A serotonin transporter gene promoter polymorphism (5-HTTLPR) and prefrontal cortical binding in major depression and suicide. *Arch Gen Psychiatry* 2000; **57:** 729–38.

Maser JD, Cloninger JD. Comorbidity of anxiety and mood disorders: introduction and overview. In: Maser JD, Cloninger CR, eds, *Comorbidity of Mood and Anxiety Disorders*. Washington, DC: American Psychiatric Press, 1990: 3–12.

Massion AO, Warshaw MG, Keller MB. Quality of life and psychiatric morbidity in panic disorder and generalized anxiety disorder. *Am J Psychiatry* 1993; **150:** 600–7.

Menin DS, Heimberg RG. The impact of comorbid mood and personality disorders in the cognitive–behavioral treatment of panic disorder. *Clin Psychol Rev* 2000; **3:** 339–57.

Mineka S, Watson D, Clark LA. Comorbidity of anxiety and unipolar mood disorders. *Annu Rev Psychol* 1998; **49:** 377–412.

Montgomery SA, Kasper S, Stein DJ et al. Citalopram 20mg, 40mg and 60mg are all effective and well tolerated compared with placebo in obsessive compulsive disorder. *Int Clin Psychopharmacol* 2001; **16:** 75–86.

Moon CAL, Jago W, Wood K et al. A double-blind comparison of sertraline and clomipramine in the treatment of major depressive disorder and associated anxiety in general practice. *J Psychopharmacol* 1994; **8:** 171–6.

Moras K, Clark LA, Katon W et al. Mixed anxiety-depression. In: Widiger TA, Frances AJ, Pincus HA, Ross R, First MB, Davis WW, eds, *DSM-IV Sourcebook*. Washington, DC: American Psychiatric Press, 1996: 623–43.

Murray CJL, Lopez AD. *Global Burden of Disease: A comprehensive assessment of mortality and morbidity from diseases, injuries and risk factors in 1990 and projected to 2020*, Vol I. Harvard: World Health Organization, 1996.

Myers JE, Thase ME: Anxiety in the patient with bipolar disorder: recognition, significance, and approaches to treatment. *Psychiatric Annals* 2000; **30:** 456–64

Nelson EC, Grant JD, Bucholz KK et al. Social phobia in a population-based female adolescent twin sample: co-morbidity and associated suicide-related symptoms. *Psychol Med* 2000; **30:** 797–804.

Nemeroff CB, Widerlov E, Bissette G et al. Elevated concentrations of CSF corticotropin-releasing factor-like immunoreactivity in depressed patients. *Science* 1984; **226:** 1342–4.

Nesse RM. Is depression an adaptation? *Arch Gen Psychiatry* 2000; **57:** 14–20.

O'Donnell D, Larocque S, Seckl JR, Meaney MJ. Postnatal handling alters glucocorticoid but not mineralocorticoid messenger RNA expression in the hippocampus of adult rats. *Mol Brain Res* 1994; **26:** 242–8.

Ormel J, Koeter MWJ, van den Brink W et al. Recognition, management, and course of anxiety and depression in general practice. *Arch Gen Psychiatry* 1991; **48:** 700–6.

Parker G. Classifying depression: Should paradigms lost be regained? *Am J Psychiatry* 2000; **157:** 1195–203.

Pawlak C, Pascual-Sanchez T, Rae P et al. Anxiety disorders, comorbidity, and suicide attempts in adolescence: A preliminary investigation. *Eur Psychiatry* 1999; **14:** 132–6.

Penava SJ, Otto MW, Pollack MH, Rosenbaum JF. Current status of pharmacotherapy for PTSD: an effect size analysis of controlled studies. *Depress Anxiety* 1997; **4:** 240–2.

Perugi G, Akiskal HS, Ramacciotti S et al. Depressive comorbidity of panic, social phobic, and obsessive–compulsive disorders re-examined: Is there a bipolar II connection. *J Psychiatr Res* 1999; **13:** 53–61.

Piaget J. *The Origins of Intelligence in Children*. New York: International Universities Press, 1952.

Pitman RK. Posttraumatic obsessive–compulsive disorder: a case study. *Compr Psychiatry* 1993; **34:** 102–7.

Post RM. Transduction of psychosocial stress into the neurobiology of recurrent affective disorder. *Am J Psychiatry* 1992; **149:** 999–1010.

Rauch SL, Baxter LR. Neuroimaging in obsessive-compulsive and related disorders. In: Jenike MA, Baer L, Minichiello WE, Eds, *Obsessive–Compulsive Disorders: Practical Management*, 3rd edn. St Louis: Mosby, 1998.

Rauch SL, Shin LM, Whalen PJ, Pitman RK. Neuroimaging and the neuroanatomy of posttraumatic stress disorder. *CNS Spectrums* 1998; **3:** 31–41.

Regier DA, Rae DS, Narrow WE et al. Prevalence of anxiety disorders and their comorbidity with mood and addictive disorders. *Br J Psychiatry* 1998; **173(suppl 34):** 24–8.

Resnick HS, Yehuda R, Pitman RK et al. Effect of previous trauma on acute plasma cortisol level following rape. *Am J Psychiatry* 1995; **152:** 1675–7.

Robins LN. How recognizing 'comorbidities' in psychopathology may lead to an improved research nosology. *Clin Psychol Sci Pract* 1994; **1:** 93–5.

Rosenblum LA, Coplan JD, Friedman S et al. Adverse early experiences affect noradrenergic and serotonergic functioning in adult primates. *Biol Psychiatry* 1994; **35:** 221–7.

Roy-Byrne P. Anxiety in primary care depression: How does it lead to poor outcomes and what can we do about it? *Gen Hosp Psychiatry* 1999; **21:** 151–3.

Roy-Byrne PP, Katon W. Generalized anxiety disorder in primary care: The precursor/modifier pathway to increased health care utilization. *J Clin Psychiatry* 1997; **58(suppl 3):** 34–8.

Roy-Byrne PP, Stang P, Wittchen H-U et al. Lifetime panic-depression comorbidity in the National Comorbidity Survey. *Br J Psychiatry* 2000; **176:** 229–35.

Rudolph RL, Entsuah R, Chitra R. A meta-analysis of the effects of venlafaxine on anxiety associated with depression. *J Clin Psychopharmacol* 1998; **18:** 136–44.

Sartorius N, Ustun TB, Lecrubier Y et al. Depression comorbid with anxiety: Results from the WHO study on psychological disorders in primary health care. *Br J Psychiatry* 1996; **S30:** 38–43.

Schaller JL, Behar D, Chamberlain T. When fluvoxamine treats only depression and clomipramine treats only obsessive–compulsive disorder – combine them? *J Neuropsych Clin Neurosci* 1998; **10:** 111–13.

Schatzberg AF, Samson JA, Rothschild AJ et al. McLean Hospital Depression Research Facility: early-onset phobic disorders and adult-onset major depression. *Br J Psychiatry* 1998; **173(suppl 34):** 29–34.

Schneier FR, Johnson J, Hornig CD et al. Social phobia; comorbidity and morbidity in an epidemiological sample. *Arch Gen Psychiatry* 1992; **49:** 282–8.

Scott S, Couser G, Schilder K et al. Postpartum anxiety and depression: Onset and morbidity in a community sample. *J Nerv Ment Dis* 1998; **186:** 420–4.

Seedat S, Lockhat R, Kaminer D et al. An open trial of citalopram in adolescents with post-traumatic stress disorder. *Int Clin Psychopharmacol* 2001; **16:** 21–5.

Segal ZV, Williams JM, Teasdale JD, Gemar M. A cognitive science perspective on kindling and episode sensitization in recurrent affective disorder. *Psychol Med* 1996; **26:** 371–80.

Shafii M, Steltz-Lenarsky J, Derrick AM, Beckner C. Comorbidity of mental disorders in the post-mortem diagnosis of completed suicide in children and adolescents. *J Affect Disord* 1988; **15:** 227–33.

Shalev AY, Freedman S, Peri T et al. Prospective study of posttraumatic stress disorder and depression following trauma. *Am J Psychiatry* 1998; **155:** 630–7.

Sherbourne CD, Wells KB, Meredith LS et al. Comorbid anxiety disorder and the functioning and well-being of chronically ill patients of general medical providers. *Arch Gen Psychiatry* 1996; **53:** 889–95.

Silverstone PH, Ravindran A. Once-daily venlafaxine extended release (XR) compared with fluoxetine in outpatients with depression and anxiety. Venlafaxine XR 360 Study Group. *J Clin Psychiatry* 1999; **60:** 22–8.

Sobin C, Sackheim HA. Psychomotor symptoms of depression. *Am J Psychiatry* 1997; **154:** 4–17.

Sonawalla SB, Spillmann MK, Kolsky AR et al. Efficacy of fluvoxamine in the treatment of major depression with comorbid anxiety disorders. *J Clin Psychiatry* 1999; **60:** 580–3.

Southwick ST, Yehuda R, Giller EL. Characterization of depression in war-related posttraumatic stress disorder. *Am J Psychiatry* 1991; **148:** 179–83.

Stein DJ: Schemas in the cognitive and clinical sciences: an integrative construct. *J Psychother Integration*, 1992; **2:** 45–63.

Stein DJ. Neurobiology of the obsessive-compulsive spectrum disorders. *Biol Psychiatry* 2000a; **47:** 296–304.

Stein DJ. *Paroxetine in pharmacotherapy of posttraumatic stress disorder.* Presented at the Biannual Congress of the Collegium Internationale Neuropsychopharmacologicum, Brussels, July, 2000b.

Stein DJ, Bouwer C. A neuro-evolutionary approach to the anxiety disorders. *J Anxiety Disord* 1997; **11:** 409–29.

Stein DJ, Hollander E. The spectrum of obsessive-compulsive related disorders. In: Hollander E, ed. *Obsessive–Compulsive Related Disorders.* Washington, DC: American Psychiatric Press, 1993.

Stein DJ, Hugo FJ. Neuropsychiatric aspects of anxiety disorders. In: Yudofsky SC, Hales RE eds, *American Psychiatric Textbook of Neuropsychiatry,* 4th Edn. Washington, DC: American Psychiatric Press, in press.

Stein DJ, Stahl S. Serotonin and anxiety: Current models. *Int Clin Psychopharmacol* 2000; **1552:** 1–6.

Stein DJ, Goodman WK, Rauch SL. The cognitive-affective neuroscience of obsessive-compulsive disorder. *Curr Psychiatry Rep* 2000; **2:** 341–6.

Stein DJ, Zungu-Dirwayi N, van der Linden GJ, Seedat S. Pharmacotherapy for posttraumatic stress disorder. *Cochrane Database of Systematic Reviews* 2000b; **4:** CD002795.

Stein MB, Chavira DA. Subtypes of social phobia and comorbidity with depression and other anxiety disorders. *J Affect Disord* 1998; **S50:** 11–16.

Stein MB, Tancer ME, Gelernter CS et al. Major depression in patients with social phobia. *Am J Psychiatry* 1990; **147:** 637–9.

Stein MB, Kirk P, Prabhu V et al. Mixed anxiety–depression in a primary-care clinic. *J Affect Disord* 1995; **34:** 79–84.

Stein MB, Liebowitz MR, Lydiard B et al. Paroxetine treatment of generalized social phobia (social anxiety disorder). *JAMA* 1998; **280:** 708–13.

Stein MB, Fyer AJ, Davidson JRT et al. Fluvoxamine treatment of social phobia (social anxiety disorder): A double-blind, placebo-controlled study. *Am J Psychiatry* 1999; **156:** 756–60.

Stuart S, Louser G, Schilder K et al. Post-partum anxiety and depression; onset and comorbidity in a community sample. *J Nerv Ment Dis* 1998; **186:** 420–4.

Sullivan GM, Coplan JD, Kent JM et al. The noradrenergic system in pathological anxiety: A focus on panic with relevance to generalized anxiety disorder. *Biol Psychiatry* 1999; **46:** 1205–18.

Tellegen A. Structures of mood and personality and their relevance to assessing anxiety, with an emphasis on self-report. In: Tuma AH, Maser J, eds, *Anxiety and the Anxiety Disorders.* Hillsdale, NJ: Erlbaum, 1985.

Tollefson GD, Souetre E, Thomander L et al. Comorbid anxious signs and symptoms in major depression: Impact on functional work capacity and comparative treatment outcomes. *Int Clin Psychopharmacol* 1993; **8:** 281–93.

van der Kolk BA, Pelcovitz D, Roth S et al. Dissociation, somatization, and affect dysregulation: the complexity of adaptation to trauma. *Am J Psychiatry* 1996; **153(suppl 7):** 83–93.

van der Linden GJH, Stein DJ, van Balkom AJ. The efficacy of the selective serotonin reuptake inhibitors for social anxiety disorder (social phobia): a meta-analysis of randomized controlled trials. *Int Clin Psychopharmacology* 2000; **1552:** 15–23.

van Praag HM, Asnis GM, Kahn RS et al: Monoamines and abnormal behavior: a multi-aminergic perspective. *Br J Psychiatry* 1990; **157:** 723–34.

van Vliet IM, den Boer JA, Westenberg HGM. Psychopharmacological treatment of social phobia; a double-blind placebo controlled study with fluvoxamine. *Psychopharmacology* 1994; **115:** 128–34.

Versiani M, Ontiveros A, Mazzotti G et al. Fluoxetine versus amitriptyline in the treatment of major depression with associated anxiety (anxious depression): A double-blind comparison. *Int Clin Psychopharmacol* 1999; **14:** 321–7.

Videbach P. PET measurements of brain glucose metabolism and blood flow in major depressive disorder: A critical review. *Acta Psychiatr Scand* 2000; **101:** 11–20.

Wittchen HU, Zhao S, Kessler RC, Eaton WW. DSM-III-R generalized anxiety disorder in the National Comorbidity Survey. *Arch Gen Psychiatry* 1994; **51:** 355–64.

Wittchen HU, Lieb R, Wunderlich U, Schuster P. Comorbidity in primary care: Presentation and consequences. *J Clin Psychiatry* 1999; **60(suppl 7):** 29–36.

Woody S, McLean PD, Taylor S, Koch WJ. Treatment of major depression in the context of panic disorder. *J Affect Disord* 1999; **53:** 163–74.

Woody SR, Taylor S, McLean PD, Koch WJ. Cognitive specificity in panic and depression: Implications for comorbidity. *Cog Ther Res* 1998; **22:** 427–33.

World Health Organization. *International Classification of Mental and Behavioural Disorders; Clinical Descriptions and diagnostic guidelines,* 10th revision. Geneva: WHO, 1992.

Yehuda R. Parental PTSD as a risk factor for PTSD. In: Yehuda R, ed. *Risk Factors for Posttraumatic Stress Disorder.* Washington, DC: American Psychiatric Press, 1999: 93–124.

Yehuda R, McFarlane AC. Conflict between current knowledge about posttraumatic stress disorder and its original conceptual basis. *Am J Psychiatry* 1995; **152:** 1705–13.

Yehuda R, Southwich SM, Nussbaum G et al. Low urinary cortisol excretion in patients with posttraumatic stress disorder. *J Nerv Ment Dis* 1990; **178:** 366–9.

Yehuda R, Giller EL, Southwick SM et al. Hypothalamic–pituitary–adrenal dysfunction in PTSD. *Biol Psychiatry* 1991; **31:** 1031–48.

Yonkers KA, Warshaw MG, Massion AO, Keller MB. Phenomenology and course of generalized anxiety disorder. *Br J Psychiatry* 1996; **168:** 308–13.

Yeragani VK, Meiri PC, Balon R et al. History of separation anxiety in patients with panic disorder and depression and normal controls. *Acta Psychiatr Scand* 1989; **79:** 550–6.

Zajecka JM. The effect of nefazodone on comorbid anxiety symptoms associated with depression: Experience in family practice and psychiatric outpatient settings. *J Clin Psychiatry* 1996; **57(suppl 2):** 10–14.

Zimmerman M, McDermut W, Mattia JI. Frequency of anxiety disorders in psychiatric outpatients with major depressive disorder. *Am J Psychiatry* 2000; **157:** 1337–40.

Zitterl W, Demal U, Aigner M et al. Naturalistic course of obsessive compulsive disorder and comorbid depression: Longitudinal results of a prospective follow-up study of 74 actively treated patients. *Psychopathology* 2000; **33:** 75–80.

Index

Abbreviations: A&D, anxiety and depression; GAD, generalized anxiety disorder; OCD, obsessive-compulsive disorder; PTSD, post-traumatic stress disorder.

Adolescents
  comorbidity in, 4
  presentation of
    depression,
    14–15
β-Adrenergic blockers, 49
Affect
  negative, 5, 5–6, 36,
    40
  positive, 5, 6, 36
Age-related change in
    presentation of
    depression,
    14–15
Agoraphobia, 16
Alarms
  evolution, 39
  false appeasement, 40
  false suffocation, 40
Amnestic disorder, 36
Amygdala, 34–6
  SSRIs and, 30
Anhedonia, 12–13
  SSRIs and, 30
Anticonvulsants, 49
Antidepressants, 45–8,
    49–52, see also
    specific types
  benzodiazepines
    combined with, 45
  newer, 46–8
    in anxiety disorders,
    49–52
    dose and duration,
    53–4
  older, 45–6
  PTSD, 22, 50, 51, 53
Antipsychotics, new
    generation, 48

Anxious arousal, 6, 36
Anxious worriers, 14
Appeasement alarm,
    false, 40
Arousal, anxious, 6, 36,
    see also
    Hyperarousal
Attentional bias in
    anxiety, 38, 39
Avoidance and
    withdrawal
  panic disorder, 16
  PTSD, 20
  social activity in
    depression, 14
  social anxiety
    disorder, 17

Basal ganglia, 32–4
Benzodiazepines, 43–5
  PTSD
    precipitated/exace
    rbated by, 22, 44
β-blockers, 49
Biology, see
    Neurobiology
Bipolar disorder,
    comorbidity of
    anxiety, 4

Children
  comorbidity in, 4
  medication, 54
  presentation of
    depression,
    14–15
  separation anxiety, 7,
    15
Citalopram, 49

Classification (diagnostic)
    systems, 1–3
Clinical features
  GAD, 22–3
  major depression,
    12–15
  OCD, 25–6
  panic disorder, 15–16
  PTSD, 19–21
  social anxiety
    disorder, 17–18
Clomipramine, OCD,
    50
Clonidine in A&D
    disorders, GH
    response to, 31
Cognitive-affective
    structures
    (schemas), 39–41
Cognitive-behavioural
    therapy, 54–5
Cognitive model,
    sequence of
    anxiety-to-
    depression, 7
Cognitive processes,
    anxiety vs
    depression, 38
Cognitive symptoms,
    depression, 13
Comorbidity, 1–11
  explanations of, 6,
    7–8, 9
  GAD and depression,
    see Generalized
    anxiety disorder
  impact, 8–10
  major depression and
    anxiety, 15

Comorbidity *continued*
  OCD and depression,
    26–7
  panic disorder and
    depression, 15
  PTSD, *see* Post-
    traumatic stress
    disorder
  sequence of comorbid
    mood and anxiety
    disorders, 6–8
  social phobia and
    depression, *see*
    Social anxiety
    disorder
Conditioning, fear, 35
Corticortico-striatal–
    thalamic–cortical
    (CSTC) circuits,
    32–4, 38
Corticotrophin-releasing
    hormone, 31–2
Course, *see* Outcome

Desipramine, OCD, 50
Development,
    neurological,
    41–2
Diagnostic and
    Statistical Manual
    of Mental
    Disorders 4th
    edition, 2, 5
Diagnostic systems, 1–3
DMS-IV, 2, 5
Dopamine blockers, 48
Drug therapy, 43–54
  dose and duration,
    53–4
  prescribing, 10

Elderly, medication, 54
Environmental factors,
    mood/anxiety
    disorders, 37
Epidemiological
    Catchment Area
    (ECA) study
  OCD and comorbid
    disorders, 27
  prevalence of A&D, 3
  sequence of comorbid
    mood and anxiety
    disorders, 7
Ethological explanations,
    sequence of
    anxiety-to-
    depression, 7
Evolution, depression in,
    39

False appeasement
    alarm, 40
False suffocation alarm,
    40
Fear conditioning, 35
Fluoxetine
  PTSD, 51
  social anxiety
    disorder, 51
Functional imaging,
    OCD, 34

Generalized anxiety
    disorder (GAD),
    22–5
  clinical features, 22–3
  comorbid with
    depression,
    23–5
  twin studies, 37
  treatment, 52, 53
Generalized social
    anxiety, 17,
    18–19
Genetic factors,
    mood/anxiety
    disorders, 37
Glucocorticoids, 31–2
Growth hormone
    response to
    clonidine in A&D
    disorders, 31

Harvard Brown Anxiety
    Research Project
    (HARP) study,
    GAD and
    depression, 23–4,
    25
Helplessness in anxiety,
    37–8
Hereditary (genetic)
    factors,
    mood/anxiety
    disorders, 37
Hippocampus, 34–6
Hopelessness in
    depression, 37
5-Hydroxytryptamine
    (and its receptors/
    pharmacology)
    see Serotonin
Hyperarousal, 5
  PTSD, 20
Hypothalamic-
    pituitary-adrenal
    axis, 31, 32

ICD-10 (International
    Classification of

Mental and
    Behavioural
    Disorders), 5
Imaging, OCD, 33–4
Imipramine
  OCD, 46
  panic disorder, 52
Inherited (genetic)
    factors,
    mood/anxiety
    disorders, 37
International
    Classification of
    Mental and
    Behavioural
    Disorders 10th
    revision, 5
Irritability, 14–15

'Kindling' hypothesis of
    recurrent
    depression, 41
Kluver-Bucy syndrome,
    36

Lithium, 49
Locus ceruleus, 31, 32

Major depression, 12–15
  clinical features,
    12–15
  comorbid with anxiety,
    15
  treatment, 53
Medication, *see* Drug
    therapy
Melancholia, 14
Memories, negative, in
    depression, 38,
    39
Midlife Development in
    the US survey,
    GAD and
    depression, 24
Monoamine oxidase
    inhibitors, 46
Mood and anxiety
    disorders
  comorbid, 4
    sequence, 6–8
  genetic and
    environmental
    factors, 37
  stressors precipitating,
    41

National Comorbidity
    Survey (NCS), 3
  GAD and depression,
    23, 24

PTSD and depression,
21
sequence of comorbid
mood and anxiety
disorders, 7
Nefazodone, panic
disorder, 52
Negative affect, 5, 5–6,
36, 40
Negative memories in
depression, 38,
39
Negative thoughts in
depression, 14
Neurobiology, 29–36
neuroanatomy, 32–6,
38–42
neurochemistry,
29–32, 38–42
neurodevelopment,
41–2
psychology and,
integration, 38–42
sequence of anxiety-
to-depression, 7
Neuroimaging, OCD,
33–4
Neuroleptics
(antipsychotics),
new generation,
48
Neurotransmitters,
29–31
Noradrenaline, 31–2
Noradrenergic and
selective
serotoninergic
antidepressants,
46
Nosology, psychiatric
(diagnostic
systems), 1–3

Obsessional slowness in
OCD, 26
Obsessive-compulsive
disorder, 25–7
clinical features, 25–6
comorbid with
depression, 26–7
neurobiology, 33–4,
36
and psychology, 38,
40
spectrum of related
disorders, 26
treatment, 27, 49–50,
53
Outcome/course/
prognosis

A&D, 8–10
GAD, 25

Panic attacks, 15–16
in social anxiety vs
panic disorder,
17–18
Panic disorder, 15–17
clinical features,
15–16
comorbid with
depression,
16–17
hypothalamic-pituitary-
adrenal axis, 31
treatment, 52, 53
Paroxetine
GAD, 52
PTSD, 51
social anxiety
disorder, 51
Pharmacotherapy, see
Drug therapy
Phobia
simple, comorbid with
depression,
temporal
relationship, 6, 7
social, see Social
anxiety disorder
Physical symptoms,
depression, 13
Positive affect, 5, 6, 36
Post-traumatic stress
disorder, 19–22
clinical features,
19–21
comorbidity, 20–1
depression, 21–2
neurobiology, 31–2
and psychology, 40,
41
treatment, see
Treatment
Prefrontal cortex, 36
Prognosis, see Outcome
Psychological factors,
37–8
neurobiology and,
integration, 38–42
Psychomotor symptoms,
depression, 13,
14
Psychotherapy, 54–5
Psychotic mood
disorders,
comorbidity of
anxiety, 4

Radiology, OCD, 33–4

Receptors and tricyclic
antidepressants,
45
Re-experiencing
symptoms
(PTSD), 20
Reversible monoamine
oxidase inhibitors,
46

Schemas, 39–41
See-saw model of
serotonin in A&D,
29–30
Selective serotonin
reuptake
inhibitors, see
Serotonin
reuptake
inhibitors,
selective
Separation anxiety, 7, 15
Serotonin (5–HT), 29
Serotonin antagonist and
reuptake
inhibitors (SARIs),
46, 47
Serotonin reuptake
inhibitors,
selective (SSRIs),
46–8, 49–52
in anxiety disorders,
49–52
children, 54
dose and duration,
53–4
efficacy across A&D
disorders, 29
elderly, 54
neurobiology/
mechanisms of
action, 30, 31, 40
Sertraline
PTSD, 51
social anxiety
disorder, 51
Social activity in
depression,
withdrawal, 14
Social anxiety disorder
(social phobia),
17–19
clinical features,
17–18
comorbid with
depression,
18–19
temporal
relationship, 6, 7
discrete, 17

generalized, 17, 18–19
neurobiology, 34, 40
treatment, *see* Treatment
Somatic anxiety, 6
Stressors precipitating mood and anxiety disorders, 41
Suffocation alarm, false, 40
Symptoms, *see* Clinical features

Temporal relationship, comorbid mood and anxiety disorders, 6–7
'Tension' disorder, 23
Therapy, *see* Treatment

Thoughts in depression, negative, 14
Tics in OCD, 26
Traumatic events (leading to PTSD and depression), 19, 21, 22, 41
Treatment, 43–55
  GAD, 52, 53
  major depression, 53
  OCD, 27, 49–50, 53
  panic disorder, 52, 53
  pharmacological, *see* Drug therapy
  psychological, 54–5
  PTSD, 44, 50, 51, 53
    early, 22
  social anxiety disorder, 50, 51, 53

early, 19
Tricyclic antidepressants, 45–6
Twin studies, major depression and GAD, 37

Venlafaxine, 46–7

WHO primary care study, prevalence of A&D, 3
Withdrawal, *see* Avoidance
World Health Organization primary care study, prevalence of A&D, 3